Deep Sleep Hypnosis

Mindfulness Meditation, Relaxation and Positive Affirmations to Fall Asleep Instantly. Start Sleeping Better, Release Stress and Overcome Anxiety

Samuel Cooper

Legal & Disclaimer

The information contained in this book and its contents is not designed to replace or take the place of any form of medical or professional advice; and is not meant to replace the need for independent medical, financial, legal or other professional advice or services, as may be required. The content and information in this book has been provided for educational and entertainment purposes only.

The content and information contained in this book has been compiled from sources deemed reliable, and it is accurate to the best of the Author's knowledge, information and belief. However, the Author cannot guarantee its accuracy and validity and cannot be held liable for any errors and/or omissions. Further, changes are periodically made to this book as and when needed. Where appropriate and/or necessary, you must consult a professional (including but not limited to your doctor, attorney, financial advisor or such other professional advisor) before using any of the suggested remedies, techniques, or information in this book.

Upon using the contents and information contained in this book, you agree to hold harmless the Author from and against any damages, costs, and expenses, including any legal fees potentially resulting from the application of any of the information provided by this book. This disclaimer applies to any loss, damages or injury caused by the use and application, whether directly or indirectly, of any advice or information presented, whether for breach of contract, tort, negligence, personal injury, criminal intent, or under any other cause of action.

You agree to accept all risks of using the information presented inside this book.

You agree that by continuing to read this book, where appropriate and/or necessary, you shall consult a professional (including but not limited to your doctor, attorney, or financial advisor or such other advisor as needed) before using any of the suggested remedies, techniques, or information in this book.

Table of Contents

Introduction

Meditation has a plethora of benefits that can help you with your most complex issues. One that you might be struggling with at the moment is the ability to fall asleep and stay asleep.

Benefits of Meditation in Your Daily Life

As individuals, the first thing that we all crave in life is – peace.

But, peace is a broad term, and one that leads to an endless list of questions.

How do we define peace?

What gives us peace?

And most importantly why do we crave it?

All of these questions are pertinent, and all of them have weight. You will begin to realize it is even more as you embark on your personal journey into the human mind, in search of it. As you seek peace however, it is important that you first try to understand how the human mind works and more importantly how meditation has multiple positive effects on the human mind, body and soul.

Meditation: A Brief History

While we think of mental health and mental development and automatically look to meditation as the perfect solution, it does beg the question - where did meditation come from? How long has it been around? Where did it originate? Interestingly, most of these questions lack a clear definitive answer even today, thousands of years since the practice was first adopted.

Some scholars have claimed that meditation, in some form or another, has existed from the beginning of humanity. However, if you are looking for a more definitive answer, India is a good place to start. In this country, most commonly associated with meditation, Vendatism has been around since 1500 BC. In China, Taoist meditation also dates back to the 5th and 6th centuries. Some scholars have dated meditation practices in the region as far back as 5,000 - 6,000 BC.

In the west, meditation didn't quite come about until the 1700s, by way of a multitude of texts on Eastern Philosophy. It wasn't until Swami Vivekananda, a Hindu monk, presented a speech at the Parliament of Religions in 1893 that this massive wave of interest in meditation brought us to where we are today.

Building Self-Awareness

For starters let's focus on self-awareness.

Take a minute and honestly ask yourself how aware you are of how your body reacts to specific situations. How do you react to light? How do you react to fear? How do you react to happy events? Take a minute and identify each of these physical manifestations of your mind and evaluate them – why do you react in this way? Have you always acted in the specific manner? What has changed, if anything?

You may notice that as you go through these questions in your mind, other questions and thoughts will enter your mind that you didn't anticipate. This is actually very typical and natural. Often times even if you think that a specific thought or specific trigger will cause your mind to think or work in a specific manner in reality it doesn't necessarily process the information in any specific way. This is why reverse psychology works on certain individuals and backfires on others – not all people react to the same form of stimulus in the exact same manner. Meditation allows you to practice introspection and truly identify how your mind reacts to specific triggers. It's almost as if your mind is doing a mental inventory of how you think, how you process, and most importantly how you react.

8

Try to think of meditation as a form of mental yoga – here the objective is to forge a stronger link between the mind and body. This is to ensure that your mind is more aware of how your body is responding specifically to cues. Meditation helps us understand our own individual sense of awareness. Helping ground us in the present moment allows us to act and think in a way that keeps us in the present.

Reducing Stress and Anxiety

This is just one benefit –meditation is not intended to simply enhance one's sense of self. In fact a major reason why so many people get involved in meditation, is because they wish to use the practice to cure themselves of unwanted stress and anxiety that they might be dealing with.

Let's simplify this, shall we?

Why do you think you are invested in meditation?

What do you feel unsure or nervous about starting your meditation program?

Try answering this instead – in the past week what are five negative things that have impacted the way you act, think and react? Make a short list in a separate journal. Have you listed them for yourself? Good! Now ask yourself how often one of these thoughts has controlled your mind. Let's say you feel unhappy at work – how often have you thought of quitting? A lot?

How often do you think about how badly you want to change jobs? Almost always?

Most importantly how often have you done something that would help you change your job, or extract yourself from that toxic work environment? Odds are you just said never very quietly under your breath. Whether or not you feel like you are ready to admit your

9

thoughts to other people, you yourself know exactly how often you are sometimes even obsessing over the negatives in your life. Do you ever wonder why you don't feel comfortable telling other people how often these negative thoughts come to your mind?

Think about it - if you don't like admitting how you are thinking, odds are that you already know, subconsciously or at some level, that what you are doing isn't good for you. Always keep in mind that while negative things will continue to happen in your life, how far you allow that negativity to spread into your personal space is a decision that you are making constantly. There is always a more productive way to deal with negative thoughts – if you feel you are stuck in a bad job, instead of obsessing over the negative features of the job entails, train your mind to focus on the way out. Line up new job interviews, consider talking to the human resources department or a supervisor; the point here is to actually actively **do** something instead of just letting things happen to you.

Taking control of the negativity that surrounds you is a key part of ensuring that you lead a healthier and happier life, because this negativity is what breeds stress and causes anxiety to build in your mind. So, if you really want to live a stress free, healthier and most importantly, happier life you are going to want to start by finding a way to reduce your stress levels, and train your mind to focus on productive activities, instead of the anxiety triggers that you have built for yourself.

Honing Mental Clarity

Another common issue many individuals tend to have to deal with is – the lack of clarity that is predominant in today's world. For the most part, research has shown that multiple mental disciplines, such as yoga and meditation, can help control the mind and even improve it. Conditions such as ADHD, which is a form of attention deficiency, have been known to show significant improvement with meditation and meditation based activities.

While it is common knowledge that physical exercise can help keep the body in shape, what people tend to forget is that the brain needs the exact same thing. Neuro exercises, or mental training activities can potentially keep our brain in shape, and can also weed out certain undesirable mental characteristics, such as depressive thoughts, or anxiety.

One of the fundamental issues currently being studied by scientists is the subject of neuroplasticity. What is neuroplasticity, you may ask? Well, simply put, scientists have begun to discover that, contrary to popular opinion, an individual's brain is not shaped at the time of their birth – in contrast the brain is actually constantly growing and learning, which is why it is possible to actually change our brains to specific forms of mental training. For example, one can retrain the brain to alter or improve multiple personality quirks, such as how attentive you are, how happy you are, how angry you are etc.

Instead of considering emotions such as happiness, or anger, or disappointment individual reactions, think of them as skills. You can train your mind so that you are more skilled at being happy or positive, although odds are you have subconsciously been training your mind to be the exact opposite. Neuroscientist Richard Davison, of the University of Wisconsin, conducted a three-month research program on the impacts of the Vipassana form of Buddhist meditation that deals with increasing mental clarity, and improving sensory awareness. On completion, he found that volunteers who had received Vipassana meditation as a form of mental training, were much faster in their ability to identify and focus on detailed information. In contrast, individuals who had not participated in the training seemed less clear and less stable in their ability to retain information. Because of this, meditation is now being seen as a form of mental exercise that helps individuals take advantage of the plasticity of the human brain, in a quantifiable and scientific manner.

Building Focus and Fortitude

However, it is not just mental clarity that is affected by meditation. In fact, a large part of meditation deals with building focus. While the science of the issue has clearly established that meditation can help enhance mental clarity by playing with the neural plasticity of the mind, it also does so on a more chemical level by releasing specific hormones to help counter your stress levels.

When you are stressed out, your body releases certain hormones to let your mind know that it is overloaded. Once your mind starts to register that you are stressed out, the body then starts to release adrenaline because it thinks that your body now needs more energy to help get you through these backlogged tasks. The only problem here is that adrenaline can work against you. While theoretically adrenaline should be helping you to get better and to do your tasks quicker and better. Adrenaline serves an important function in our bodies, but unless we learn to control stress, adrenaline works against us. Instead of helping us get through stressful moments, excessive adrenaline instead increases anxiety, and multiplies our stress reaction.

Keep in mind the release of adrenaline in your body is a physical reaction to fear or danger, or some sort of immediate desperate need – this is a physical reaction, that has been passed on to us from our ancestors, who at the time needed that extra bit of energy to fend off predators or to stay alive. Now imagine having that level of pressure put on you every single day, because you are unable to distinguish between a life-and-death situation, and a workplace crisis. Your body simply doesn't know the difference.

This of course is where meditation steps in. Meditation gives us a sense of self worth and power, so that when we are faced with a challenge, we are not immediately dropping the ball and going into "danger" mode – instead we are calmly teaching ourselves to cope, which in turn allows our brain to focus and develop better coping strategies.

Have you ever given yourself a social media detox? Is your immediate reaction after you wake up to check Facebook? One of the first things you might want to do is slowly detach from your phone or the distractions of social media over the next seven days.

Meditation teaches your brain to do the exact same thing in terms of the topics on which you are focusing. By slowly teaching yourself to focus on the factors which you would like, such as positive outcomes, you simultaneously build your mental fortitude. You're training your brain to not go into panic mode at the slightest thing. At the same time, you are also teaching yourself how to react to those smaller, yet persistent mental problems that you find yourself facing on a daily basis. Win-win!

Emotional Intelligence

So, what else does meditation help with? Well, for starters, it is also an extremely important tool in the development of emotional intelligence. As you begin to become more aware of your own self and how you react to specific situations, you will also realize that you are attuned to how people around you react to those same situations. This form of awareness is also commonly known as emotional intelligence, and is currently considered to be of extremely high value. Indeed, some scientists have begun to prefer the evaluation of emotional intelligence over the evaluation of one intelligence quotient to determine a person's potential.

While you probably ask yourselves multiple times whether or not you are good enough or smart enough, odds are you probably don't ask yourself if you are compassionate enough or if you are a good listener. If you are familiar with the television program, The Big Bang Theory, you've probably seen that the protagonist Sheldon Cooper has been portrayed to be an individual with extremely high IQ, but extraordinarily low EQ factor. In later seasons, this impacts his career growth, as well as his personal life. This is actually extremely common - no matter how smart you are, in order to truly succeed in life, you will find that you will require a certain amount of emotional intelligence.

Start asking yourself the following questions to gauge what your emotional intelligence levels are:

1. Are you generally a calm person? Are you capable of maintaining this calm in stressful situations?

2. Would you consider yourself to be compassionate? Are you well attuned to the needs of others?

3. In your opinion, do you have a tendency to make good decisions?

4. Are you capable of listening to what other people have to say? Do you take people's opinion into consideration?

5. Do you believe that you have a positive influence on the people around you?

6. Are you an impulsive person? How impulsive do you consider yourself to be, on a scale of 1 to 10?

7. What is your standard mind-set – happy or sad?

Were the answers that you just provided generally negative in nature? If so odds are you have a low EQ, the good news is it doesn't really matter how low your EQ is, because you can actually build on your EQ levels through meditation. The act of meditation not only helps you detach from negative thoughts, it is also known to help you assess and attune yourself to the emotions of other people. Poker players for instance are known to have extremely high emotional intelligence levels; their advanced emotional intelligence is what allows them to 'read' emotions such as fear or hesitation in their opponents, which in turn enables them to make better plays.

But, most importantly, your emotional intelligence levels will help you deal with years of emotional baggage that have burdened your inner mind control. Gone are the days that you couldn't control your temper. With the help of meditation, you can now actively deal with your anxiety, your depression, and your negative thought patterns, replacing them with solid reasoning skills and problem-solving capabilities.

Relaxing the Mind

And finally, one of the least appreciated and yet possibly one of the most beneficial attributes of meditation – mental relaxation. Think about it...when was the last time you gave your brain a break. Keep in mind that going away on holiday does not count. When was the last time that you sat still for 15 minutes and did absolutely nothing. You didn't mentally list the tasks that you have to do, you didn't make decisions about what you're going to need for dinner. You didn't worry about ten different things that happened today – you literally did nothing.

Let's be honest, odds are it's been a while. Lucky for you, meditation is actually known to trigger the relaxation response in the mind, which means that any time you spend meditating is time you are spending allowing your brain to go into a state of absolute relaxation.

Why is this important? The more relaxed your brain is the easier it is for you to fall asleep, to manage your stress levels, and to reduce your anxiety. Think of it as your emotional balance, by relaxing your brain you are training it to maintain better emotional equilibrium, which in turn allows you to become a more balanced individual.

These are just some of the numerous benefits that are attached to meditation. Meditation is also known to enhance kindness in societies, and help individuals become more community minded. It also plays a strong role in fighting addictions; studies have shown that recovering alcoholics generally do much better when they receive meditative training. So, with all our doubts put to rest, the only question now is how do we do it, or more accurately how do we prepare for it?

Don't worry, we have you covered – keep scrolling!

Chapter 1. - What is hypnosis?

These guided meditations are going to be in the "I" voice. You will want to imagine these thoughts going through your head as if they were your own thoughts. If you want, you could always listen to these and repeat afterwards out loud or record your own voice to help you really get into these kinds of hypnosis. Make sure you are sitting somewhere comfortable and safe for each of these.

The first one will be great to do while you are preparing for bed. It will help to get you in the right mindset needed to really become sleepy. It is a relaxing way to free your mind of the anxious thoughts that might have been there all day.

The second one is going to help you fall asleep even faster than the first one. You can pair them together perfectly for a restful night's sleep, or you can try them at different moments to see which works best for you.

Meditation for Winding Down and Getting Sleepy

For this meditation, make sure that you start by ensuring that you are focused on getting into a sleepy place and are completely comfortable in bed. Ensure that no distractions are around and that you've finished up all of your nighttime routines. Put your phone somewhere that it will not be distracting and make the light and the music right.

To get into this meditation, make sure that you are keeping your eyes closed and focused only on falling asleep. For the remainder of the meditation, we are going to use "I" statements. Remember to think of these thoughts as they come into your mind as if they were your own. As we count down from ten, make sure to focus on your breathing, and making your body as relaxed as possible.

Ten, nine, eight, seven, six, five, four, three, two, one.

I can feel my body get lighter and lighter as I relax my muscles and melt into the bed. I can tell that my body is tired and needs to be relaxed at this point. It is important that I nestle myself into bed so that I can better get the rest I need to start the day off tomorrow.

As I start to become more and more relaxed, I feel like my bed is turning into a cloud. Each breath I let out, I feel myself relaxing more and more. The air that I breathe in is energy that's going to help me feel even more relaxed.

As I breathe in, I feel all of the things that happened to me today, but as I breathe out, I let these thoughts go and pay no more attention to them. As I'm breathing in, I accept all that has happened to me today, and as I breathe out, I let go, knowing that holding onto it is only going to cause me more stress.

With every breath that I let out, I feel lighter and lighter. Each time I let the breath out, I feel like I'm sinking deeper into the clouds. I know now that I do not have to carry all of the weight with me that I have been feeling throughout the day.

I can become more and more relaxed, letting myself float and become lighter and lighter. I am drifting away from my bed now, being lifted away like a big fluffy cloud. I am not afraid of anything that I might be leaving behind. I know that it is okay to drift up and away, into the sky and looking down below me.

I am drifting from all of my responsibilities. I do not have to take care of them now. They'll be there when I get back. Right now, I only need to focus on drifting into the sky and becoming relaxed. The only thing that I need to think about is becoming more tired, feeling the fluffy cloud around me that keeps me nice and cozy.

I start to float up higher and can see the things that are below me. All around there are people tired, trying to get to sleep just as I am. There are some people walking down the street. Maybe they're walking home. There are other people driving. Maybe they're driving home.

Maybe these people are going into work. Maybe they have responsibilities that they need to take care of tonight. I do not. I do not have anything that I need to worry about. I have done my work for the day, and it doesn't really matter what's waiting for me tomorrow.

Worrying about the things that I have to do later is not going to help me feel any better now.

I worry about these things too much, and it makes it harder for me to fall asleep. I know now that the only thing I need to worry about is drifting away.

I do not need to really worry about this, however. It is not a pressing issue. I might not be asleep, but at least I am resting my body.

As I look down, I see all of the people that aren't yet resting theirs. They could be in bed, but they chose to be out late. They could be drifting in the clouds, sleepy like me, but instead they are staying awake, making it harder for themselves to think and function throughout the day tomorrow.

I am taking care of my health. I am looking out for myself tomorrow. By making sure that I am focused on relaxing and falling asleep, I am ensuring that tomorrow will be an easy day for me. Tomorrow I will be relaxed, because I'm making sure that I'm tired now.

Sometimes, it is hard for me to fall asleep because I do not spend enough time winding down. It can take a little longer to get fully relaxed, and I need to remember that as I'm trying to fall asleep. It will be easier for me now to fall asleep because I am paying special attention to really winding down.

I can feel my body becoming more and more relaxed as I regulate my breathing.

As I am floating above on my fluffy cloud, I can see the wind ripple through the tree leaves. I can feel that air blow through my hair, travelling gently into my lungs. As I take a big deep breath in, I can feel how this air fills me with so much relaxation. I let the wind out slowly, and I become one with the world around me. Though not everyone is asleep, I can still feel the peace and serenity that exists all throughout this beautiful sky.

As I continue to let the air enter and exit my body, I get higher and higher. Before I know it, I can see the clouds around me, making pure gray surroundings. Some stars are still twinkling through the clouds, and I can see the black night sky behind them. As I look down, I see less and less as I become enveloped within the cloud.

Where I am now, I can no longer see the cloud that I'm actually lying on. Where my original cloud starts and stops is no longer easily identifiable. I have become one with all of the clouds at this point.

I am still floating, not worried about what's going on below me.

There is nothing around, and I feel that relaxation in every part of my body. It has never been easier than it is now to completely relax and focus only on this moment.

I can twist and move my body a bit and that will change where and how I am travelling throughout the sky. I have no plan for where I'm going, however. It doesn't really matter if I go forward, backward, left or right. The only thing I care about is feeling every last ounce of my body relax.

It is not until now, when I'm up in the clouds, that I really realize just how much tension I carry throughout my body.

Now that I am here, nowhere, nothing around me but clouds, I realize that I can feel like this all the time.

Never before have I been so tired, and now I am ultimately relaxed so I can get a full and deep night's sleep.

The more that I practice going up into the clouds like this, the easier it will be to fall asleep on a regular basis. I can do this when I'm napping, if I wake up in the middle of the night, or simply when I initially try to fall asleep.

I understand now how important it is going to be for me moving forward to ensure that I am fully relaxed before going to sleep. If I'm not tired but need to go to sleep, it can be harder for me to actually drift away.

If I want to ensure that I can fall asleep easily and stay asleep, I need to relax my entire body.

The cloud is starting to drift down now, and I understand what it means to completely let go of everything that I am feeling and allow myself to become more rested.

The cloud is passing over the streets now, and I can see that so many people are focused on getting back into bed. My cloud is moving towards my house, doing all the work so that I can remain as still and calm as possible. I do not have to worry about doing anything other than becoming entirely asleep.

My cloud gently puts me back into my bed. I can feel the warm blankets around me and the soft mattress beneath me. Everything that I experienced throughout the day is over now, and I do not have to worry about doing anything other than drifting away. Everything that stressed me out is over, and what waits tomorrow is beyond anything I can predict.

As I count down from ten, I will be able to either drift asleep, or stay tired enough to move onto the next meditation. I can still feel my eyes become heavier, my breathing slower. When I reach one, I will be almost all the way asleep.

Ten, nine, eight, seven, six, five, four, three, two, one.

At times, life has the unfortunate tendency of feeling like a constant battle. Similarly, as experienced by all living things, there are times when we become tired and unable to constantly face things. It is at times like this that we are tempted to give up or to surrender ourselves to the unknown - not because we believe in a greater power steering our way, but because no matter what we do, it seems as if we can't help but fall constantly.

Every time we fall down seems to be one time too many, and our ability to stand up again seems to gradually erode itself. Strength, courage, and motivation all seem to elude us.

This is where the promotion of inner strength comes in. Contrary to popular opinion, inner strength isn't something that is simply within us, but rather it is built and rebuilt constantly over the years. One of the best ways to fortify your inner strength so that you can overcome the tangible and intangible obstacles that have come your way is by teaching yourself how to promote that inner strength and rebuild your sense of being able to do something.

Are you ready? Amazing! Here we go.

Meditative Guide to Promote Inner Strength

Before we begin with our guided meditation, however, it is important for you to ensure you are the best physical position. Strength meditations require solace and solitude, which is why you are going to want to find yourself a quiet and safe space where you can begin. For this specific exercise, try sitting upright in such a manner that you maintain a perfect line from the back of your neck to the base of your spine. Hard backed chairs or strong surfaces are recommended. Both the lotus, half lotus, and upright seated position may be adopted as per your convenience.

Once you have found your position, look around yourself, and stretch beforehand, lowering yourself into the chosen position and slowly closing your eyes to begin. As you close your eyes, direct your focus solely onto your breathing, feel the long indrawn breath travel through your body, and release the air from your lungs.

You are now ready to start your meditative guide.

Breathe deeply, and as you do so, allow your eyes to slowly close.

As you breathe, you can feel the energy start to flow through your body, drawn in through your mouth and then traveling from the top of your head to the tips of your toes. A glowing violet light of energy seems to cascade through your being.

Allow your back to relax and slowly start to follow this guiding light.

Start by feeling the powerful force in your mouth, and then see it travel downward to your Dantien. Your Dantien is the core of your being, positioned just an inch-and-a-half above your belly button. It is from here that the soft purple light is radiating throughout your body.

Focus intently on your shoulders; carefully start by allowing your left shoulder to relax and release the tense self-doubt it carries.

As you feel your left shoulder unburden itself, turn your attention to your right to do the same.

The present moment surrounds you. You are unburdened. You are light.

Understand that in this moment you are free of inabilities.

There is nothing the present moment withholds from you.

There is nothing you cannot do in this present moment.

The present moment simply exists.

Along with it, you will find a soft persistent strength glow dimly in the background.

This soft purple light, is your core – it is your strength.

Visualize yourself in your mind's eye.

As the light covers you, notice that underneath the violet light, a pulsing red energy is coating your body. This is your power source and your passionate ability to do whatever needs to be done.

You are invincible.

You are extremely powerful.

This power is buzzing around you, sinking in and out of your very being to allow you to step forward and harness your choices to its infinite abilities.

Breath.

Relax.

You are capable of all things, and there is nothing that you cannot do.

Collect your self-doubt, and surrender it to this pulsating being, and as you do, notice that the thick deep red that was pulsating around you seems to be shifting to a softer color.

Soft blue light rains down on your inner self.

In your mind's eye, reach out and feel them.

These are hopeful positive rays of light being showered upon you.

As they touch your passionate red energy, your energy changes to the bright violet that you once saw.

You are strong.

You are capable.

As a person, you have already overcome great odds. Mentally, who are you, and what have you overcome to become who you are?

Identify, your fears and how and why they have scared you.

Envision yourself overcoming them.

Breathe deeply.

Release.

Remind yourself that there is nothing in this world or beyond it that prevents you from having all that you desire. You are capable and worthy.

There is nothing you cannot do, and there is nothing you will not achieve.

Time is your friend.

You are talented and proficient.

Your abilities are limitless.

You have a gift of attaining, and you will attain all that you desire and more.

Focus on your breathing.

As you do, notice the way the air flows from your soul.

Breathe in.

Release.

Remember that today you are capable of attaining all your goals. Your goals are not limited by any failures that you may perceive. You are whole, and you are capable.

Repeat this with your soul: 'Today I am strong and capable. My capabilities are not confined by my failures. My future is infinite. I am infinite.'

Breathe in carefully to the count of five, and as you exhale, slowly open your eyes and recognize your present self.

You are strong and capable, and there is nothing you cannot do. There are no obstacles you can't overcome.

Guided Meditation to Improve Insomnia

One of the major mental health problems dealt with today happens to be the unfortunate lack of sleep caused by insomnia.

Insomnia itself stems from a variety of response states, including anxiety and worry. The anxiety state leads to your body being put in a state of constant alert all day, which, in turn, causes the body to deteriorate quickly and be forced to fight off tiredness and difficulty breathing, as hyperventilation weakens the body's physical strength reserves.

The worry state is similar in that it results in a physical stress on your mind by replaying the fears or uncomfortable images you have had which, in turn, make sleep or restfulness impossible. The worst part about the worry state, however, is not just that it keeps you from being comfortable, but rather the way in which it seeps into your daily life. With anxiety and worry being a regular part of life, insomnia also tends to follow.

So, let's tackle our insomnia before it digs its roots in any deeper, shall we?

Meditative Guide for Insomnia

As before, try to use the first five minutes of this exercise to find yourself a comfortable position from which you can conduct the meditation. Keep in mind that unlike other forms of meditation, insomnia meditation cannot be conducted in a seated position, meaning that you will want to find yourself a comfortable bed or position from which you can continue.

It is also important that you keep in mind that insomnia meditations are not to be undertaken while you are in control of any form of vehicle or heavy machinery. Strong bright lights are considered inadvisable and should be turned off for the best results.

You are now ready to start your meditative guide.

Breathe deeply three times and purge your body of stress.

As you breathe in each time, hold your breath to the count of four and release slowly.

Breathe in.

Release.

Breathe in.

Release.

Breathe in.

Release.

Your objective today is to teach yourself how to fall asleep and to relax. Over time, you may have forgotten how to fall asleep and how to release the stronghold you have on your unconsciousness so that you can allow your mind to recharge.

We will be counting backward from fifty, and by the time we reach zero, you will have mastered your ability to slip into calm, relaxed unconsciousness.

Start by asking yourself why you are having such a difficult time falling asleep.

Is there a specific thought that is worrying you?

Is there a list of things that you need to get done?

Is there a prospective outcome that you are nervous about?

Whatever it is that is keeping your mind constantly engaged, I want you to take a minute and truly focus on it.

Ask yourself if there is anything for you to do now, in this moment.

Breathe in.

Release.

You'll notice that, despite the fact that there is nothing to do at this moment, your consciousness is finding it difficult to release this particular thought.

Empty your mind's eye and open a blank sheet of paper. Mentally type up the problems and the fears that you have, which are constantly breaking through your consciousness. Here, you are downloading your worries and your fears so that they are no longer grasping on to your mind.

Once you are done, close the document, and refresh your mind.

You are clear.

You are unburdened.

You are light.

Your thoughts and worries are there and will remain there for you to return to tomorrow. For now, you are meant to focus only on your own consciousness.

Breathe in.

Release.

Breathe in.

Release.

Breathe in.

Release.

Today, you choose to be unburdened and, in turn, you feel that choice free you of the heavy weight that is upon your shoulders.

Remember that today, you are free, you are not tied down, and you are not fettered.

You have the ability to feel the tension in your neck and shoulders slowly release as you allow yourself to sink comfortably into the arms of relaxation.

Feel relaxation sink deeper into your bones and radiate from your spine and your ribs, all the way down to your toes. Every part of your body is releasing energy, and as you slowly continue to release it, you are allowing the comfortable cradle of sleep to rock you into a melodic lull.

Repeat the following with your soul: 'Today, I choose relax. My goal today is to release the tension from my body and to free myself from all forms of awareness.'

Breathe deeply to the count of four, and as you breathe out, allow the weight of your consciousness to lower your eyelids.

You are falling deeper and deeper into your unconsciousness.

Breathe in.

Release.

Breathe in.

Release.

Breathe in.

Release.

Guided Meditation to Positive Consciousness

The subconscious mind is generally put off balance by two major issues, the first being fear and the latter being worry or the re-living of fear in conscious moments with conscious thoughts. In order, therefore, to cleanse the soul of all forms of negative reenactments, we have chosen to push forward with what is called guided meditation on positive consciousness.

Paths of consciousness are all intertwined. As you grow older, you will begin to realize that each of these paths underpins your actions by filtering the energy with which you choose to process your life's force. As such, the best way to rebuild your bridge to relaxation is to work on a positive filter through with you can view your own self and transform your consciousness while also healing and moving forward.

Meditative Guide for Positive Consciousness

As one of the simplest forms of meditation, positive consciousness works almost exclusively on the rebuilding of conscious mind maps. For whatever reason, at some point in your life, your self-esteem, your self-confidence, and your courage to move forward have all been tampered with.

By focusing on positive consciousness, you can attempt to see all these self-inflicted wounds. No longer are your thoughts at the mercy of other people's perceptions of you. In contrast, you will now become whoever it is that you need to be in order to meet your own demands and aspirations. As you seek a suitable position to begin this meditation, stretch out your body to first rid it of any wasteful energy that has been left over from the day before.

As you seat yourself, stretch out your back until you feel a sharp pull, and at this point, lower your neck to be level with the floor. Outstretch your arms upon the tops of your knees and lift your palms upward and leave them facing toward you.

You are now ready to start your meditative guide.

As you slowly close your eyes, fix within your mind's eye a point from which you are meant to gather all consciousness. Remember that your consciousness has suffered in recent days and, as such, is in need of healing. By promoting positive consciousness, not only are you rebuilding this broken stream of good will, but you are fortifying it so that it will be protected from any future harm.

Breathe in carefully to the count of five.

Hold to the count of four and then slowly release.

You are resilient.

You are calm.

You are undisturbed.

You are gifted.

Exhale deeply, purging yourself of all the negative stress and energy that has been building in your body, and instead, open your mind's eye and with it, you should be able to see and feel the energies around you.

You are seeking within yourself a way in which you can let go and be at peace.

The cool darkness behind your eyes is inviting you to feel calm and at peace. The bright lights at the periphery of your mind are showing you the endless possibilities that you have at your disposal.

I am capable.

I am smart.

I am efficient.

I am worthy.

I am talented.

I am resourceful.

I am bright.

I am attentive.

As you remind yourself of these things, open your mind once again to see the various energies that are flowing through your being. With your mind, start to follow each individual channel of energy until you can see how they flow beautifully into each other.

This time, as you repeat each positive affirmation, weave it through one of the strands of energy so that it will flow perfectly though your mind from now on and forever after.

I am capable.

I am smart.

I am efficient.

I am worthy.

I am talented.

I am resourceful.

I am bright.

I am attentive.

Each of these thoughts is now an inviolable part of your consciousness. As your energy begins to build in your center, allow it to move upward to your mind and, as you raise your neck, lift your face forward to accept the new revolutionary truths that have become a part of your reality.

You are powerful.

You are significant.

You are respected.

You are loved.

Repeat the last four phrases in your mind once again.

I am powerful.

I am significant.

I am respected.

I am loved.

Breathe in.

Release.

Breathe in.

Release.

Breathe in.

Release.

As you prepare yourself to open your eyes, you are embodying a positively minded individual.

Chapter 2. - Principles for self-hypnosis for sleep

For this meditation, make sure that you have become relaxed enough to fall asleep. You will instantly fall asleep at the end, so you must ensure you are in a safe and comfortable place. Complete pitch-black darkness is preferred, but if you must sleep with a light on, ensure that it is dim. You can include a noise machine or sound effects machine as well if that will help you become more relaxed.

As I count down from ten, start to let your body feel free and focus on hearing the thoughts that I say as if they were your own.

Ten, nine, eight, seven, six, five, four, three, two, one.

I am feeling more and more relaxed right now.

There is nothing around me.

I am alone, and this is OK. I see nothing but pitch black and darkness. As an image starts to burn into my vision, I quickly dissolve it.

I start to focus on nothing. No thoughts from the previous day are coming into my brain.

Each time I start to think about something that causes me stress, I focus only on nothing.

There is nothing to focus on, but that is enough to keep me distracted from anything that might keep me awake.

As an image burns into my vision again, I push it away. There are no images that I will see that will keep me distracted long enough.

My vision is trying to make something out in front of me, but that is just how my eyes work.

They are so tired now, so I need to keep my lids closed so that I can fall asleep.

All day, my eyes are looking at different things around me. Sometimes I have to squint to see things in the distance, and other things are in plain sight.

Sometimes I look past the things I do not want to see, and other times I move my vision away fast when I'm sneaking a peek and do not want others to know.

My eyes are tired now, so I need to rest them. I have so much left to see as I go throughout my day. I do not need to see anything right now. I need to keep these eyes focused on rejuvenation.

My eyes are done for the day, just as my mind is. When I start to think about what I have to do tomorrow, I push that thought away. Nothing that I will encounter is something that I need to be stressed about right now.

I am prepared. I am ready. I will conquer, and I will succeed. Right now, I need to focus on getting very deep sleep.

Though I can hear some things in the background, it is all silent in my mind. I hear nothing but what is going on around me right now.

Each sound is one that pushes me further and further to sleep. It is like a piano lullaby that slowly lulls me to a drowsy stupor.

I feel the nothingness throughout my body. The lack of sight and sound and everything else around me makes me feel so much lighter.

When my body is free, my mind is free. When my mind is free, my body is free.

When I can be relaxed, it will be so much easier to fall asleep.

I will not even have any nightmares or other vivid dreams to keep me up. There will be nothing to prevent me from going to sleep, and I will get exactly the right amount of sleep.

I realize now that there is nothing around me. Everything is black. Everything is dark. Everything is far.

This does not scare me. This fills me with peace. This reminds me that I have nothing to worry about. I have nothing to think about. I have nothing to do.

The only thing I need to focus on right now is myself. I am focused on my breathing.

I am tired, and I am starting to fall asleep. This is exactly what my body needs.

This nothingness, this black state of space is the perfect solution to my need for a deeper sleep. This is what will bring me closer to being rejuvenated and refreshed tomorrow.

I feel nothing above me, next to me, below me, or around me. It is just me, and my mind. I can feel my eyes, I can feel my breathing, and I can feel my head. All of these are perfectly relaxed, helping me to focus on what is more important than anything in this world right now – falling asleep.

As nothing surrounds me, I become more aware of my breathing. I can feel the air fill my lungs and leave through my body.

Air is always around me. This will always soothe me. The only thing I need is air. Whether I am trying to wake up or fall asleep quicker, air is what will help me. It is my body's rhythm. When I am breathing, I am creating something. I have created life within me.

I can feel the air enter my body now. It comes in slowly as I start to fall asleep. Even though I am trying to get a deeper sleep, I need to make sure my breathing is right.

If I fall asleep without regulating my breathing, it can keep me from getting a deep sleep.

I breathe in for five as I feel the air come into my body. I breathe out again for five more as it exits.

Breathe in. One. Two. Three. Four. Five.

I hold it for a moment, feeling it spread relaxation from my chest to my fingers, and down to my toes.

I breathe out for one, two, three, four, five.

I continue to do this, each time, my breathing getting a little slower and slower. This is helping me to relax, become calm, and feel my body become air itself.

I am not someone who needs to be working right now.

I am not someone who needs to be anxious right now.

I am not someone who needs to be awake right now.

I need to go to sleep, and my breathing, and my eyes, and my mind, and everything else around me is going to help me fall asleep. I am doing exactly what needs to be done right now, and it will help me get a good night's sleep that I thoroughly deserve. I am focused on nothing but giving my body the exact thing that it needs to power me through tomorrow.

I can spend my night worrying, my sleep dreaming of the future, and my morning anxious about waking up. None of this will help me do better tomorrow, however. What is going to be the most beneficial to me includes getting a good night's sleep and repowering my body for what is to come tomorrow.

I can feel my eyes getting heavier and my breathing getting slower.

There is still nothing around me, and that doesn't scare me. There is no one that is going to hurt me, and not a soul will disturb my peaceful slumber.

I am not above ground or below it. I am the air that exists everywhere. I am drifting into the nighttime sleep that everyone else is in right now. The only thing that matters is that I feel this sleep heavily.

The biggest concern I have at the moment involves falling asleep.

Even if I do not fall into a heavy slumber at first, that's fine. I am relaxing my body, giving it the rest that it needs to carry me throughout the day.

When my sleep is right, so is everything else. Even if I am getting to sleep too late, any sleep is better than none at all.

When I focus on getting deep sleep, it helps me to get the most out of my time as I lay unconscious.

I still feel my body expanding into the dark space around me, my sight getting deeper and deeper. Each time something passes in my mind, I let it drift off without giving it a second thought.

If I feel like there is something to be afraid of, I remember that is not the case. I am safe. I am focused. I am not afraid. I am not anxious. I am not stressed.

Each time something pops into my vision and wants to take my mind's energy, I push it out. Everything dissolves around me into the blackness.

That is where I am going now. Into the dark. There is no turning back for today. I will wake up tomorrow, ready and energized. As I count down from twenty, I continue to breathe in for five, and out for five.

Chapter 3. - Induction techniques to get self-hypnosis

At this point in the audio, I invite you to make yourself as comfortable as possible in your bed. Please have all the light's turned off and distractions put away. You have already put in a full, hard day of work. Think of sleeping sound and comfortable through the night as a reward for working so hard.

How was your day today?
Were you productive?
How did you feel?

I want you to think about these questions as you settle further into the bed. Gently tuck yourself under the cover, and we will begin our journey. Ready?

Inhale deeply. Hold onto that breath for a moment, and then let it go. To begin, I am going to lead you through an induction script for self-hypnosis. By allowing yourself to slip into this state of mind, it will help you let go of any stress you may be holding onto, even if it is in your subconscious. I am going to help you tap into these emotions so you can let them go and sleep like you never have before.

All of us are stressed. Honestly, who can sleep when they are worried? In this state of mind, you probably feel too alert to even think about sleeping. When you are stressed, the adrenal glands in your body release adrenaline and cortisol. Both of these hormones keep you awake and stop you from falling asleep.

In the audio to follow, we will go over letting go of your worries, even if it is just for the night. You are in a safe place right now. Anything you need to get done can wait until tomorrow. It is important you take this time for yourself. We all need a break from our responsibilities at some point or another. I invite you now to take another deep breath so we can focus on what is important right now; sleep.

To start, I would like you to close your eyes gently. As you do this, wiggle slightly until your body feels comfortable in your bed. When you find your most comfortable position, it is time to begin breathing.

As you focus on your breath, remind yourself to breathe slow and deep. Feel as the air fills your lungs and release it in a comfortable way. Feel as your body relaxes further under the sheets. You begin to feel a warm glow, wrapping your whole body in a comfortable blanket.

Before you let go into a deep hypnotic state, listen carefully to the words I am saying at this moment.

Everything is going to happen automatically.

At this moment, there is nothing you need to focus on. You will have no control over what happens next in our session. But you are okay with that. At this moment, you are warm and safe. You are preparing your body for a full night's rest and letting go of any thoughts you may have. There is no need to think of the future or the past. The only thing that matters right now is your comfort, your breath, and the incredible sleep you are about to experience.

Now, feel as the muscles around your eyes begin to relax. I invite you to continue breathing deeply and bring your attention to your eyes. They are beginning to feel heavy and relaxed. Your eyes worked hard for you today. They watched as you worked, they kept you safe as you walked around, and they showed other people you were paying attention to them as you spoke. Thank your eyes at this moment and allow them to rest for the night so they will be prepared for tomorrow.

Your breath is coming easy and free now. Soon, you will enter a hypnotic trance with no effort. This trance will be deep, peaceful, and safe. There is nothing for your conscious mind to do at this moment.

There are no activities you need to complete. Allow for your subconscious mind to take over and do the work for you.

This trance will come automatically. Soon, you will feel like you are dreaming. Allow yourself to relax and give in to my voice. All you need to focus on is my voice.

You are doing wonderfully. Without noticing, you have already changed your rate of breath. You are breathing easy and free. There is no thought involved. Your body knows exactly what you need to do, and you can relax further into your subconscious mind.

Now, you are beginning to show signs of drifting off into this peaceful hypnotic trance. I invite you to enjoy the sensations as your subconscious mind takes over and listens to the words I am speaking to you. It is slowly becoming less important for you to listen to me. Your subconscious listens, even as I begin to whisper.

You are drifting further and further away. You are becoming more relaxed and more comfortable. At this moment, nothing is bothering you. Your inner mind is listening to me, and you are beginning to realize that you don't care about slipping into a deep trance.

This peaceful state allows you to be comfortable and relaxed. Being hypnotized is pleasant and enjoyable. This is beginning to feel natural for you. Each time I hypnotize you, it becomes more enjoyable than the time before.

You will enjoy these sensations. You are comfortable. You are peaceful. You are completely calm.

As we progress through the relaxing exercises, you will learn something new about yourself. You are working gently to develop your own sleep techniques without even knowing you are developing them in the first place.

On the count of three, you are going to slip completely into your subconscious state. When I say the number three, your brain is going to take over, and you will find yourself in the forest. This forest is peaceful, calm, and serene. It is safe and comfortable, much like your bed at this moment.

As you inhale, try to bring more oxygen into your body with nice, deep breaths. As you exhale, feel as your body relaxes more and more into the bed. Breathing comes easy and free for you. As you continue to focus on your breath, you are becoming more peaceful and calmer without even realizing it.

As we continue, you do not care how relaxed you are. You are happy in the state of mind. You do not have a care in the world. Your subconscious mind is always aware of the words I am saying to you. As we go along, it is becoming less important for you to listen to my voice.

Your inner mind is receiving everything I tell you. Your conscious mind is relaxed and peaceful. As you find your own peace of mind, we will begin to explore this forest you have found yourself in, together.

Now, I want you to imagine you are laying near a stream in this beautiful and peaceful forest. It is a sunny, warm summer day. As you lay comfortably in the grass beside this stream, you feel a warm breeze, gently moving through your hair. Inhale deep and experience how fresh and clean this air is. Inhale again and exhale. Listen carefully as the stream flows beside you. A quiet whoosh noise, filling your ears and relaxing you even further.

It is becoming less and less important for you to listen to me. Your subconscious mind takes hold and listens to everything I am saying. All you need to do is enjoy the beautiful nature around you. The sunlight shines through the trees and kisses your skin gently. The birds begin to sing a happy tune. You smile, feeling yourself become one with nature.

Each time you exhale, I want to imagine your whole body relaxing more. You are becoming more at ease. As you do this, I want you to begin to use your imagination. You are lying on the grass. It is located in a green meadow with the sun shining down on you. The sun is not hot, but a comfortable warm.

Imagine that there are beautiful flowers blooming everywhere around you. Watch as the flowers move gently in the breeze. Their scents waft toward your nose as you inhale deeply and exhale.

When you are ready, I want you to imagine that you begin to stand up. As you do this, you look over your left shoulder gently, and you see a mountain near the edge of the beautiful meadow. You decide that you would like to take a trip up to the top of the mountain to see this beautiful view from a different angle.

As you begin to walk, you follow the stream. Imagine gently bending over and placing your hand not the cool, rushing water. As you look upon the water, imagine how clean and cool this water is. The stream flows gently across your fingers and it relaxes you.

When you are ready, we will head toward the mountain again. As you grow closer to the mountain, the birds begin to chirp. Inhale deep and imagine how the pine trees smell around you. Soon, you begin to climb the mountain at a comfortable pace.

You are enjoying the trip. It is wonderful to be outside with this beautiful nature, taking in all the sights and sounds. Now, you are already halfway up the mountain. The meadow grows smaller as you climb higher, but you are not afraid. The scene is beautiful from up here, and you are happy at this moment.

As you reach the top, take a deep breath and give yourself a pat on the back for your accomplishment. Take a look down on the meadow and see how small the trees look.

The breeze is blowing your hair around gently, and the sun continues to shine down on the top of your head. Imagine that you are taking a seat at the very top of the mountain. You close your eyes in your mind's eye and take a few moments to appreciate this nature. You wish you could always be this relaxed.

When you take your life into your own hands, you will be able to. This is why we are here. Of course, you may be here because you want to sleep, but you can't do that truly unless you learn how to let go of your stress. Through guided meditation and exercises within this audio, you will learn how to become a better version of yourself. I am here to help you every step of the way.

Soon, we will work on deepening your trance. You are beginning to relax further into the meditation and are opening your heart and soul to the practice. Remember that you are safe, and you are happy to be here.

Chapter 4. - Before bed hypnosis

In order for us to dive deeper into your subconscious, I will need you to relax as much as you can. In the following few minutes, we are going to try a muscle relaxation exercise. As I mention an area, I invite you to focus on the area, so you can tense and relax it. When I tell you to tense an area, this should not cause you any pain whatsoever. If at any point you feel discomfort, please stop or try to ease up on tensing the area.

When you are ready, take a deep breath. Inhale...exhale...and we will begin.

We are first going to start with your neck and your shoulders.

To start, please try to raise your shoulders up toward your ears. As you do this, you will feel the muscles in your neck and shoulders begin to tighten. Feel the tension, where it builds, and then release. Allow your shoulders to drop to their normal position. Your shoulders and neck should feel comfortable. If not, try this again until you feel the muscles release and relax.

Remember to breathe through this process. Inhale...and exhale. Good.

Now, we will move onto your hands.

I want you to squeeze both hands into fists. Your hands are in very tight balls. You can try to pretend that you are squeezing a rubber ball. Hold this ball in your hands and feel as the tension begins to build first in your hands, and gently moves up your forearms.

When you feel the pressure, release your hands. Gently shake them and get rid of any tension. How do your hands feel now? They should feel much more relaxed.

With your neck and hands relaxed, let us draw your attention to your forehead. Our faces do a lot of activity for us through the day. Our facial expressions allow us to tell people when we are happy, sad, or stressed. I want you to raise your eyebrows. Feel as the muscles in your forehead begin to tighten and hold that position. Now, try to lower your eyebrows and tighten your eyes. Hold this tight for a few moments and then release.

Notice now how relaxed and smooth your forehead feels now that you have released the tension. Your eyelids are gently resting over your eyes, and you feel comfortable again. When you are ready, inhale…exhale…now move your focus to your jaw.

If you can, tightly close your mouth. Feel how tight your jaw feels as you clamp it closed. Your lips are tense across your teeth, and the tension builds in your jaw. Take a moment to note how this feels, and then relax your jaw. Allow your mouth to fall relaxed and loose. Release all tension and feel how wonderful and light your head feels.

To complete your relaxation, we will now practice deep breathing. Deep breathing is an excellent practice as it can help cure any stress or anxiety you may be feeling at any given moment. As you breathe, you remind your body that this is a fundament to your survival. Any time we are stressed, you may not notice, but our breathing patterns change. By doing this, it is your body's attempt to survive physical activity.

While helpful in actual dangerous situations, it won't help you if you are anxious over something that is isn't dangerous to you immediately. When our breathing becomes rapid, it also becomes shallow. Short, shallow breaths may make you feel like you are unable to catch your breath. This is because you are not breathing properly.

When we do not breathe properly, your lungs fill with stale, old air. This is not helpful as new air is unable to enter. In this sense, you need oxygen to fill yourself with positive energy. Proper breathing techniques will help you in multiple ways from relaxing to letting go of stress. When you learn to breathe the right way, you can stop the negative cycle and gain the ability to calm your body under stressful circumstances.

If you find yourself breathing too quickly, it could cause tingling, numbness, or even lightheadedness. The cure here is to learn how to slow down your breathing. Bring your focus on keeping your breath deep and full.

Now, I am going to go through a breathing exercise with you. Before we begin, I want you to take careful note of how you are breathing right now. Are your lungs full? Do you feel like you have old air stuck in there? Are your breaths quick or long?

When you are ready, I want you to inhale slowly and count to four…We will pause and count to three…and then exhale to the count of five. Ready?

Wonderful. Let us try it a few more times. Truly try to focus on each step of your breath. Trust the natural rhythm of your breathing to help relieve any anxiety or stress you may be holding onto.

With your breath in mind, it is now time to give in completely to relaxation. It is time to assure your body and mind are both set for the session. Now, I want you to repeat after me, and then we will begin.

I am gently going into a state of total relaxation

(Pause)

At this moment, my body and mind are both relaxing.

(Pause)

I am going deeper and deeper. I am relaxing deeper and deeper.

(Pause)

Every muscle in my body is relaxing. I feel peaceful. Everything around me is quiet.

(Pause)

Wonderful. Now, I am going to count from the number one to the number ten. When I reach ten, your whole body will be relaxed. You will be safe and completely calm in your mind and in your soul. When you are ready, take a deep breath, exhale, and we will begin.

One…feel as all of the muscles in your face begin to relax. You are releasing the tension from your forehead. The muscles around your eyes soften. You allow your jaw to go slack. Your face was active all day long. At this moment, it is time to give your face a rest.

Two…the muscles in your neck begin to melt. They are loosening and relaxing. Your neck worked all day to keep your head on straight. Feel as the muscles relax and melt into your pillow and bed. They can finally rest up for another day.

Three…Feel as your shoulders relax further into the bed. If there is any tension in them, shake them out gently and allow them to fall away from your ears. Many of us hold our shoulders scrunched up through the day. We do it subconsciously when we are scared, stressed, or even just cold. Allow your shoulders to relax completely and feel them fall peacefully onto the bed without a care in the world.

Four…Gently bring your focus to your hands. They are finally done for the day. They held your food for you, typed away on the computer, and held your loved one. Now, they are free of any responsibility. Give them a quick flex and relax your hands. Allow your fingers to fall away from your fists and allow them to rest wherever they are at this moment.

Five…as the rest of your body begins to rest, feel as your chest muscles relax. They follow suit from your neck and your shoulders.

Focus on the lungs inside of your chest. Breathing is coming easily and naturally. Each time you breathe, you feel yourself relax further into your meditation. Peacefully, thank your lungs for doing such a wonderful job to support you.

Six...imagine the muscles in your back begin to loosen. As you lay in bed, they are finally able to relax. They worked hard all day to keep you upright and supported you when you needed them most. Now, they can relax and enjoy a good night's rest. Feel as the muscles in your back and lower back let go of any final tension.

Seven...now, the muscles in your stomach are relaxing. If you were stressed today, you might have felt a lot of tension in your stomach. This is why we use the expressions "butterflies in my stomach" or "I felt sick to my stomach." There are many connections between our psyche and our stomachs. At this moment, you have no worries. Your stomach can relax and rest for the night.

Eight...feel the muscles of your buttock begin to relax. This is a location many of us don't spend a lot of time thinking about. Feel as the muscles loosen and relax. Your buttock sinks deeper into the bed, and you feel yourself becoming even more comfortable as your body gets ready for a full night's rest.

Nine...the top of your thighs is relaxing. Your legs do so much work through the day. They allow you to walk from place to place and support you. Gently release any tension that may be built up in your legs and picture them sinking deeper and more comfortable into the bed.

Ten...finally, feel like the muscles in your lower legs relax. Your feet let go of all tension, and you find yourself completely comfortable. There is not a single place in your body holding onto tension. You feel comfortable, safe, and at peace.

Now, you are in a state of total and deep relaxation. From the top of your head to the tip of your toes, you are totally relaxed.

You are feeling better and better. You are ready to focus on sleep at the count of three.

One...

Two...

Three...

Chapter 5. - Mindfulness meditation to fall asleep

If you feel any of these areas tensing up, focus your attention here. Breathe in…and breathe out…choose to relax and soften these areas. As you breathe, imagine the air bringing total relaxation to these areas and allow the tension to leave your body. I invite you to continue this pattern until your breathing becomes deep and slow again.

Notice now how your body has become more relaxed than it was before. Feel as your muscles sink into the bed as you relax further and deeper. Your jaw is becoming loose. Your mouth is resting, and your teeth are slightly apart. Now, your neck is relaxing, and your shoulders are falling away. Allow this to happen and let your muscles become soft.

I want you to return to your safe place. Imagine that this place is spacious, comfortable, and filled with a positive light. In this place, you have nothing to worry about, and you have all the time in the world to focus on yourself.

In this safe place, I want you to imagine the sun streaming in. The light fills you with warm and positive emotion. Thee are windows where you can see the beautiful nature outside. Your space can be wherever you want it to be. It can be by the mountains, by the ocean, or perhaps even on a golf course.

Return your focus back on your safe place. Imagine how warm and comfortable the room is. Walk over toward the comfortable bed and imagine how wonderful it feels to sink into the sheets. The sun is shining down on you, and you feel relaxed and warm. The bed is so soft around you, and you feel so at peace at this moment.

Notice now how these peaceful thoughts begin to fill your mind. They are filling your conscious and are clear. Any other thoughts you had before are drifting away. Your mind is falling into a positive place as you feel yourself drifting away. The space around you is safe and peaceful, and beautiful.

Any other thoughts you have at this moment, pass through your mind and drift off like clouds drifting by. Allow these thoughts to pass without judgment. There is no sense in dwelling on them when you are in such a safe place. All you have at this moment is peace and quiet.

Any time a worried thought arises, you turn your focus back to your safe place. In this location, you can get rid of any stress you may have on a daily basis. You are here to relax and enjoy this moment. There is nothing that can bother you. You are free from stress and responsibilities here.

When you are ready, you feel your body begin to drift off to sleep. You are beginning to slip deeper and deeper toward the land of dreams. As you feel your attention drift, you are becoming sleepier, but you chose to focus on counting with me. As we count, you will become more relaxed as each number passes through.

We will now take a few breaths, and then I will count from the number one to the number ten. As you relax, your mind will drift off to a deep and refreshing sleep. Ready?

Breathe in…one…two…three…and out…two…three.

Breathe in…one…two…three…and out…two…three.

Breathe in…one…two…three…and out…two…three.

Wonderful. Now, count slowly with me…one…bring your focus to the number one

Two…you are feeling more relaxed…you are calm and peaceful…you are drifting deeper and deeper toward a wonderful night of rest.

Three…gently feel as all of the tension leaves your body. There is nothing but total relaxation filling your mind and your body. At this moment, your only focus is on quietly counting numbers with me.

Four…picture the number in your mind's eye. You are feeling even more relaxed and at peace. Your legs and arms are falling pleasantly heavy. You are so relaxed. Your body is ready for sleep.

Five…you are drifting deeper. The sleep begins to wash over you. You are at peace. You are safe. You are warm and comfortable.

Six…so relaxed…drifting off slowly…

Seven…your mind and body are completely at peace. You have not felt this calm in a while…

Eight…everything is pleasant. Your body feels heavy with sleep.

Nine…allow your mind to drift…everything is floating, and relaxing…your eyelids feel comfortable and heavy…your mind giving in to the thought of sleep.

Ten…you are completely relaxed, and at peace…soon, you will be drifting off to a deep and comfortable sleep.

Now that you are ready to sleep, I will now count from the number one to the number five. All I want you to do is listen gently to the words I am saying. When I say the number five, you will drift out of hypnosis and sleep comfortably through the night.

In the morning, you will wake up feeling well rested and stress-free. You have worked on many incredible skills during this session. You should be proud of the hard work you have put in. Now, it is time to sleep so you can wake up in the morning feeling refreshed.

Chapter 6. - Positive affirmations for better sleep

An affirmation is an affirming statement that you make to yourself in order to reiterate the importance of an idea. Throughout the day, you might think of negative affirmations that validate your perspective. These can include things like, "I'm not good enough," or "Nothing is going right in my life." These statements aren't necessarily the whole truth, but they might have a certain element that can help solidify one perspective.

These affirmations are going to help you focus on what's most important and remember the ideas needed in order to get your best night's sleep possible. Repeat these back to yourself, write them down and make notes around your home, or simply remember them in your mind when you need them the most.

Affirmations for Falling and Staying Asleep

The best way to include these affirmations in your life is to repeat them daily. They will help retrain your brain to think more positively rather than the negative ways that you might be thinking now.

In order to reiterate the importance of affirmations, including physical activity can help you to remember them even more. When you integrate a physical exercise with a mental thought, it helps make it more real. It will be easier to accept these affirmations in your life when an emphasis is put on truly believing them.

The first movement that you can do in order to remember these exercises is to physically hold an item. It can be something as small as a stone that you keep in your pocket, or you can pick out a special pillow or blanket that you choose to use with each affirmation that we list throughout the following sections.

As you are saying these affirmations, physically touch and hold these items. Let it remind you of reality. Stay focused and grounded on remembering the most important aspects of these affirmations.

Alternatively, try implementing new breathing exercises that we haven't tried yet. The method of breathing in through your nose and out through your mouth is important, but as we go further, there are other ways that you can include healthy breathing with these positive sleep affirmations.

One method is by breathing through alternate nostrils. Make a fist with your right hand with your thumb and pinky sticking out. Take your pinky and place it on your left nostril, closing it so that you can only breathe through one.

Now, breathing for five counts through that nostril.

Then, take your right thumb, and place it on your right nostril, closing that and releasing your pinky from the other nostril. Now, breathe out for five.

You will notice that doing this breathing exercise on its own is enough to help you be more relaxed. Now, when you pair it with the affirmation that we're about to read aloud, you will start to put more of an emphasis on creating thinking patterns around these affirmations.

An alternate method of breathing is to breathe in for three counts, say the affirmation, and then breathe out for three counts. You can do this on your own with the affirmations that are most important to your life.

It will be beneficial for you to have a journal that you keep affirmations in as well. Have one handy to write these affirmations down as they apply to your life. Writing about them will help you remember them and keep a note of the things that are most effective in your life.

When you are having a bad day, you can visit these affirmations. When you need a little confidence booster, or some motivation, use these affirmations.

We will now get into the reading of these. Remember to focus on your breathing as we take you through these, and if you are not planning on drifting off to sleep once they have finished, taking notes can help as well.

Healthy Sleep Dedication

1. I am dedicated to making healthy choices for my sleeping habits.

2. The things that I do throughout my day will affect how I sleep; therefore, I am going to make sure to focus on making the best choices for all aspects of my health.

3. I will do things that aren't always easy because it will be in the best interest of my health overall.

4. When I am well-rested, everything else in my life become easier.

5. I am more focused when I have slept an entire night, so I know that falling asleep is incredibly important to my health.

6. Developing healthy habits is easy when I dedicate my time towards a better future.

7. It feels good to take care of myself.

8. I deserve a good night's sleep; therefore, I deserve everything else that will come along with this benefit.

9. I am naturally supposed to get rest. It is not wrong for me to be tired and to choose to do healthy things for my sleep cycles.

10. Dreams are normal, and I am focused on embracing them and avoiding nightmares.

11.   I choose to go to bed at a decent time at night because it is best for my health.

12.   Whatever is waiting for me tomorrow will still be there whether I get a full night's sleep or not, so it is best to ensure I am getting the proper amount of rest.

13.   I take care of my body because I know that it is the only one that I will ever have.

14.   I allow discipline in my life to guide me in the right direction to make the choices that are healthiest for my individual and specific lifestyle.

15.   I nourish my body and make sure I get the right amount of nutrients to keep me energized throughout the day.

16.   I am strong because I get the right amount of sleep.

17.   Getting the right kind of sleep is good for my mental health.

18.   I am happier when I am well-rested. I am in a better mood and can laugh more easily when I have had a good night's sleep.

19.   I am grateful for my opportunity to be healthier and to get better sleep.

20.   I am thankful that I have the ability to make the right choices for my health and overall well-being.

21.   Having habits is not a bad thing, I just need to make sure that my habits are healthy ones.

22.   I am less stressed out when I am able to get a better night's sleep.

23.   I am the best version of myself when I am healthy. I am healthiest when I am well-rested and focused on getting a better night's sleep.

24.   Everything else in my life will fall into place as I focus on getting the best night's sleep possible.

25.   I love myself, therefore I am going to put an emphasis on dedication to better sleeping habits so that I can feel better all the time.

Relaxing

1. I am feeling relaxed.

1. Relaxation is a feeling I can elicit, not a state that I have to be in depending on certain restrictions.

2. I can feel the relaxation in my mind first and foremost.

3. As I feel my body becoming relaxed, I can feel that serenity pass through the upper half of my body.

4. All of the tension that I might have built throughout the day is now starting to fade away.

5. I am focused on myself and centered within my body.

6. I can tell that my muscles are becoming more and more relaxed.

7. There is nothing that is concerning me at the moment.

8. There will always be stressors in my life, but right now, I do not have to worry about any of those.

9. As I focus on being calmer, it is easier for my mind to relax.

10.   I do not have to be afraid of what happened in the past.

11.   I cannot change the things that are already written in history.

12.   I don't need to be fearful of the future.

13.   I can make assumptions, but my predictions will not always be accurate.

14.   I can focus on the now, which is the most important thing to do.

15.   As I start to draw my attention to the present moment, I find it easier to relax.

16.   The more relaxed I am, the easier it will be for me to fall asleep.

17.   The faster I fall asleep, the more rest that I can get.

18.   I have no concern over what is going on around me. The only thing I am concerned with is being relaxed in the present moment.

19.   I exude relaxation and peace. Others will notice how quiet, calm, and collected I can be.

20.   I am balanced in my stress and pleasure aspects, meaning that I have less anxiety.

21.   I am not afraid of being stressed.

22.   Stress helps me remember what is most important in my life.

23.   Stress keeps me focused on my goals.

24.   I do not let this stress consume me.

25.   I manage my stress in healthy and productive ways.

26.   I have the main control over the stress that I feel. No one else is in charge of my feelings.

27.   It is normal for me to be peaceful.

28.   I allow this lifestyle to take over every aspect, making it easier to have a more relaxed sleep.

29.   When I can truly calm myself down all the way, it will be easier to stay asleep.

30.   I let go of my anxiety because it serves me no purpose.

31.   I am excited for the future.

32.   I am not afraid of any of the challenges that I might face.

33.   It is easy for me to be more and more relaxed.

34.   There is nothing more freeing than realizing that I do not have to be anxious over certain aspects in my life.

35.   I will sleep easier and more peacefully knowing that there is nothing in this world that I need to be afraid of.

Staying Asleep

1. Nothing feels better than crawling into my bed after a long day.

2. My bedroom is filled with peace and serenity. I have no trouble drifting off to sleep.

3. Everything in my room helps me to be more relaxed.

4. I feel safe and at peace knowing that I am protected in my room.

5. I have no trouble falling asleep once I am able to close my eyes and focus on my breathing.

6. I make sure all of my anxieties are gone so that I can fall asleep easier.

7. When bad thoughts come into my head, I know how to push them away so that I can focus instead on getting a better night's sleep.

8. I am centered on reality, which involves getting the best sleep possible.

9. It is so refreshing to wake up after a night of rest that was uninterrupted.

10.   Any time that I might wake up, I have no trouble knowing how to get myself back to sleep.

11.   Whenever I wake up, it is easy to get out of bed within the first few times that my alarm clock rings.

12.   The better night's sleep I get, the easier it is for me to wake up.

13.   I release all of the times that I have had a restless night's sleep.

14.   No matter how many times I have struggled with my sleep in the past, I know that I am capable of getting the best night's sleep possible.

15.   My sleep history doesn't matter now. I want to get a good night's sleep, so I will.

16.   The more I focus on falling and staying asleep, the fresher I will feel in the morning.

17.   Getting a good night's sleep helps me look better as well. My hair is bouncier, my face is fresher, my eyes are wider, and my smile is bigger.

18.   Sleep is something that I need.

19.   Sleep is something that I deserve.

20.   No matter how little work I got done in a day, or how much more I might have to do the next day, I need to get sleep.

21.   There is no point in my life where sleep would be entirely bad for me. It's like drinking water. I could always at least use a little bit of it.

22.   I am alert when I am focused on sleeping better.

23.   It is easier to remember the important things I need to keep stored in my memory when I have been able to have a full night's sleep.

24.   I can focus on what is going on around me more when I have been able to sleep through the night.

25.   There is nothing about getting sleep that is bad for me. As long as I am doing it in a healthy way, it will improve my life.

26.   I know how to cut out bad sleeping habits.

27.   I understand what is important to start doing to get a better sleep.

28.   As soon as I start to lay down, I am focused on drifting away.

29.   I do not let anxious thoughts keep me awake anymore.

30.   I will sleep healthy from here on out because I know that it is one of the most important decisions for my health that I can make.

25 Affirmations to Help You Find Happiness

1. Every individual person has the right to happiness – and so do I.

2. I deserve to be healthy, happy, and whole no matter where I am. Happiness is a right that I am entitled to, and nothing can take that right away from me.

3. My happiness is not measured by what other people see, but by how I feel.

4. I am consciously choosing to allow happiness to take over my mind and my soul, and I am ridding my soul of pain and hardship.

5. I do not want to be anyone but myself, and as I move to be a better version of myself, I am hoping to be a stronger and better version of me.

6. Happiness and love are two parts of my soul; I am happy and my happiness is filled with love.

7. Other people's thoughts do not influence my happiness. My happiness is my own - I am its owner, and I alone am its master.

8. Today, I choose to be happy. Happiness is a choice. Happiness is a possibility.

9. I am worthy of being loved, and my worth brings me joy and happiness.

10. I choose my experiences, and my experiences are what shape my happiness. I am joyful and whole.

11. It is more important to me that I feel happy and am happy than that I look or appear to be happy to the outside world.

12. I am giving myself permission to be a happy person. I can now be the happiest version of myself.

13. I choose to put gratitude and joy in front of fear and insecurities. I seek to be whoever I wish to be, because that will bring me happiness.

14. I am happy because my actions today allowed me to be cheerful and genuine. My actions are a reflection of my soul, and my soul is happy.

15. I find it impossible to be negative. Negativity does not attract me or speak to me. I am happy and content in being me.

16. I choose to be happy for the people around me. When the people around me are doing well, they are making me happy.

17. For me, happiness is a journey; it is a destination which I am seeking constantly.

18. My happiness is made up of the memories of the people I love.

19. Making other people happy makes me happy and, as such, I am a happy person.

20. I am a happy virus, and my hope is to spread happiness and joy wherever I go.

21. The entire concept of living is the concept that brings me joy. I am happy because I am alive, and I live everyday happier than I was yesterday.

22. Happiness comes to me naturally, and because of these happy thoughts, I am always in a happy state of mind.

23. My future is bright and happy, because I have chosen my future to be bright and happy.

24. I choose to randomly perform acts of kindness. I believe that kindness breeds happiness, and I choose to be happy.

25. I am happy and I am enough.

25 Affirmations to Relieve Anxiety

1. I'm not afraid of fear. Fear does not control me. In fact, fear is merely a reaction.

2. I choose consciously to let go of my past worries and to move forward into the good and the light that await me.

3. I am strong and capable. I grow stronger with every breath I take, and every time I exhale, my fears leave me.

4. I reject failure, and I choose to fill my mind and soul with only positive nurturing thoughts.

5. I believe that I can, and, therefore, I believe if not today, tomorrow I will succeed.

6. I am like a magnet. I repel negativity and negative thoughts in all forms.

7. I do not make mistakes, but rather I learn lessons - and from every lesson I have learned more and more.

8. I am willing to invest in my power to change my life by releasing the anxiety that holds me back.

9. I am stronger than I may seem.

10. My fears and my depression do not control who I am or who I am going to be.

11. I am on a constant journey to discover a more calm and peaceful version of me.

12. I have made it through this far, and I will make it through until the end.

13. I belong exactly where I am. I am not unwanted or ugly – I am perfection.

14. I celebrate everything that has to do with me, because I am madly in love with myself and all that I can be.

15. I will love myself enough to get through this moment.

16. I choose to feel safe and secure, even when the darkness comes in.

17. Anxiety is a real problem, but I am a real solution and my mind is stronger than anxiety's grip on it.

18. Anxiety does not control me; it merely shows me where not to go and what not to do.

19. Anxiety is merely the fear of the unknown, and I am an explorer who is ready to know everything.

20. I have survived this far, and I will survive as long as I want.

21. I am someone who is capable of looking beyond the pain that has been inflicted upon me, because pain does not matter, and what I choose to do does matter.

22. I am whole despite my anxiety.

23. My anxiety cannot control me, because I do not allow it to be in the driving seat.

24. I have everything I need to be the best version of me.

25. I am always in charge of my own mind, l, and my mind does not choose to be anxious.

1. Meditation 1: Body Scan

Wiggle, wiggle, wiggle until you find a comfy position in your bed... great job!

Now, gently let your eyelids get heavy and close.

We're going to take some deep breaths together. Breathing in through the nose and out through the mouth.

To get ready, blow all your air out [*Make blowing noise*]

And in through the nose

2

3

4

And out through the mouth

2

3

4

5

6

In through the nose

2

3

4

And out through the mouth

2

3

4

5

6

In through the nose

2

3

4

And out through the mouth

2

3

4

5

6

And one more more! In through the nose

2

3

4

And out through the mouth

2

3

4

5

6

...

Let your breath return to normal and start to notice the relaxing position you are in.

For this meditation, we are going to take a journey together to scan different parts of your body and observe anything you might be able to feel.

All you have to do is relax and follow along with my voice.

First, just start to notice your breath. Maybe paying attention to the coolness at your nostrils when you breathe in. Or how your tummy moves up and down with each breath.

...

Notice how easy is to breath in... and out as you relax more and more.

...

As you inhale, your tummy fills up like a balloon.

And as you exhale, the balloon lets it's air out.

...

Feel the cool air coming in through your nostrils, traveling down your throat, and filling up your belly.

...

Feel your chest and stomach growing as you breathe in and falling when you breathe out.

...

Notice the tiny moment right between each in breath and out breath.

...

There is nothing to do right now, but keep your attention on your breath. Wherever you notice your breathing the most.

...

...

Now bring your attention to the tip top of your head.

Notice any sensations you may have there. You might have to really relax and be a detective to notice anything at all on the top of your head.

...

Now, moving your attention to your forehead. Imagining a tiny steamroller smoothing out your forehead and letting all the tiny muscles there completely melt away.

...

Moving down to your eyes, your cheeks, your mouth, and your jaw. Noticing any holding or squeezing in places around your eyes completely relax.

...

Now, bring your attention to your shoulders. Letting your shoulders fall away from your ears as they start to get heavier and heavier. Imagining that your shoulders are two block of ice, just melting into water.

....

With every exhale, relaxing and allowing the muscles in the shoulder to melt away.

...

Now, bring your attention to your arms, your elbows... what tiny feelings can you notice in your arms and elbows? Maybe coolness or heat? Maybe even the feel of the sheets or your pajamas touching the arms and elbows.

And now down to your forearms and wrists... then to your hands... and all the way through your fingers to the very tips of your fingers...

71

Notice the weight of your arms. Do they feel heavy like a boulder or light like a feather?

Noticing the length of the arms. Have you ever payed attention to how long your arms are?

Take a few moments here to notice any sensations in your arms, hands, and fingers.

…

As you soften and relax your hands with each breath, you might even begin to notice a slight buzzing or tingling sensation in the fingers. Just tuning in to anything you can feel in your hands.

…

Now, move your attention up to your chest and the area around your heart.

Pay attention to your heartbeat. Just noticing what's there for you right now?

…

Can you sense the beating of your heartbeat? If you'd like - I invite you to place one of your hands over your heart and see if you can feel your heartbeat.

…

Just continuing to breathe gently and listening to your heartbeat.

...

Now, using your next few in breaths to gently fill up your belly like a balloon.

What do you notice in your belly? Can you notice the release of the belly when you breathe out?

...

Allow yourself to be a curious observer.

...

Now, move your attention down to your hips.

Notice the tops of your legs... notice your knees... notice your calves... notice your shins

And all the way down to your ankles... your feet... and through the very tips of your toes...

...

Just seeing if you can notice any slight feelings of aliveness in your feet.

...

And now gently bringing your attention back to your breath.

...

With each exhale, you feel your whole body relax and melt into the bed. Sensing and feeling your entire body at once.

...

Every breath makes you feel more at ease and relaxed.

...

Allow yourself to drift. Into a deep, restful, sleep.

2. Meditation 2: Breathe to Sleep

Wiggle, wiggle, wiggle until you find a comfy position in your bed... great job!

Now, if you haven't already, gently let your eyelids get heavy and close.

We're going to take some deep breaths together. Breathing in through the nose to the count of four and out through the mouth to the count of six.

To get ready, blow all your air out [*Make blowing noise*]

And take deep breath in through the nose...

2

3

4

And out through the mouth...

2

3

4

5

6

Again breathing in through the nose…

2

3

4

And out...

2

3

4

5

6

In…

2

3

4

And out...

2

3

4

5

6

See if you can keep counting your breaths just like that.

Breathing in for four... and breathing out for six.

...

If your mind runs away in thought or you lose count of the breath, that's okay! Just gently return your attention to the breath.

...

Each time you breathe out, imagine all the tiny muscles in your forehead and around your eyes smoothing out and melting away.

...

Let your jaw relax open and your tongue rest on the bottom of the mouth like it has it's own little bed there. Completely softening the jaw, the mouth and the tongue.

...

Still breathing in for the count of 4 and out for 6. If that ever feels uncomfortable, you are more than welcome to continue breathing normally and just follow along with my voice.

...

Letting your shoulders melt away from your ears. Maybe even imagining that your shoulders are blocks of ice melting away into water.

...

Letting your stomach relax as you notice it gently filling up like a balloon with each in breath, and letting go with each out breath.

...

Noticing all the places where your body is touching the bed...

Is it cool there or warm? Can you feel pressure, heaviness, or lightness? Just noticing whatever is there for you.

...

And now as your feet and toes completely relax, you might begin to notice a slight buzzing or tingling sensation there.

...

Pretending your feet are completely asleep, taking a little foot nap. Notice how much more you can feel when you relax the feet more and more.

...

If you haven't done so already, just let you breath return to normal. Not worrying about counting or changing it any way.

...

Now, I am going to ask you to use your imagination!

If you were painting a picture of yourself breathing, and you had to choose what color to paint your breath, what color would it be? Would it be red like a dragon's fire or blue like a cool ocean breeze? Just take a moment to pick a color for your breath. Go with whatever color comes to your mind first.

And now with every in breath, imagine that color pouring in through the bottoms of your feet, traveling up your body, and all the way to the tip top of your head.

On each outbreath, sending the colorful breath back down through your body and back out the bottoms of your feet.

Just continue imagining your colorful breath rising and falling. All the way up to your head on the in breath, and all the way out through the feet on the out breath. Rising and falling like gentle waves in the ocean.

…

Continue breathing the air up to your head... and out through your feet on the exhale. Imagining the color you chose traveling up and down your body.

…

It's perfectly okay if you get distracted or start thinking about something else. Just notice that your mind has wandered away, and gently come back to imagining the rise and fall of your colorful breath.

…

Imagining every inch of your body being completely softened and relaxed when the color of your breath touches it.

…

If you start to drift off, that's perfectly fine. You can just allow my voice to become a background noise as you continue to breathe.

…

For the next minute or two, just completely relax with nothing to do.

Allow your breathing to be just as it is. Allow your body to be just as it is.

Nothing to do.

...

Relaxing and letting go… into a calm, peaceful sleep.

Meditation 3: 5 Senses Meditation

Wiggle, wiggle, wiggle until you find your most comfy position in your bed!

Now, if you haven't already, allow your eyelids to start to close.

We're going to start by taking a few breaths together. Breathing in through the nose to the count of four and out through the mouth to the count of six.

To get ready, blow all your air out [*Make blowing noise*]

Deep breath in through the nose…

2

3

4

And out through the mouth...

2

3

4

5

6

In through the nose…

2

3

4

And out...

2

3

4

5

6

In…

2

3

4

And out...

2

3

4

5

6

Now just let your breath return to normal - not forcing it or changing it in any way. Just noticing your breath.

…

Listen to your breath like you would listen to a close friend who is telling you a secret.

...

We are going to use all of our five senses today to help us relax and fall asleep. The five senses are seeing, hearing, smelling, touching, and tasting.

Allowing you breathing to return to normal, let's begin our journey through the five senses.

With your eyes remaining gently closed, notice what you are seeing!

Even though your eyes are closed, you might be able to name a color that you are seeing on the inside of your eyelids- like pink, or blue, or black. Notice how you might be able to see tiny amounts of light - even with your eyes still closed!

What do the inside of your eyelids look like?

You might experiment with allowing your eyelids to open just a sliver on each in breath, then fall closed again on each outbreath. Feeling the weight of your eyelids becoming heavier and heavier with each out breath.

...

Let all the tiny muscles around the eyes soften and relax - just see whatever you are seeing.

...

Now, start to notice any sounds that are around you.

What can you hear?

Maybe noises in the room nearby?

 Maybe far away noises that you can only hear if you listen closely...

...

As you continue to listen very carefully, you might begin to notice the sound of your own breathing.

...

What does your breath sound like? Some people say that the breath of a sleeping person can sound like gentle ocean waves.

...

Just continuing to notice whatever sounds come up. Seeing if you can pinpoint the moment when each sound begins and the moment when each sound ends.

...

Isn't it relaxing to just listen?

...

Now, begin to notice what you can smell.

If you don't smell anything, just notice the coolness of the air on the tips of your nostril each time you breathe in. Then releasing and letting go with each out-breath.

...

Continuing to breathe and smell anything you can.

…

If you get lost in thought, no problem! Just gently return you attention back to the cool air at the tips of your nostrils.

…

...

Taking a moment to notice all the places where your body touches the bed. And now all the places where your body touches the sheets or your pajamas.

Feel the weight of your arms and legs as they melt away and sink into the bed.

...

If you tune in closely to your hands and fingers, you might even notice some small feelings of aliveness there. Maybe a little buzzing or tingling. Softening and relaxing your hands more and more might even allow you to feel this aliveness even more.

...

If there's any feeling in your body that's calling your attention, let yourself observe it. If it's a nice feeling, just label it: "nice feeling". If it's a bad feeling: just calmly label that too: "bad feeling".

...

Listening with your whole body to the sensations of touch.

...

And now tasting whatever you can taste. Maybe noticing any leftover tastes from something you ate or the taste of your toothpaste if you recently brushed your teeth. If you don't taste anything, what does nothing taste like?

...

Noticing how your body is a bit field of sensations. From sights, to sounds, to smells, to sounds, to tastes, things continue to enter in and out of your attention.

...

Let's finish our meditation by taking a few relaxing breaths together. In through the nose to four, and out through the mouth to six.

In...

2

3

4

Out...

2

3

4

5

6

Repeat 4 more times.

And now letting your whole body be limp and heavy like a noodle. Nothing to do right now except relax... and slowly drifting... into a deep, deep sleep.

Chapter 7. - Visualizing your path through meditation

While meditation can be undertaken just about anywhere at just about any given time, there are certain guidelines that you need to follow if you want your meditation to be as effective as possible. However, keep in mind that meditation is meant to be flexible. The idea is not to create a rigid system that you will find difficult to follow. Meditation is meant to be easy and modifiable to adjust it to meet your specific needs.

Attuning to Physical Sensations

The physical world around you impacts your mind. This is a fact that we are all aware. What we don't necessarily notice is that just as the physical world impacts our mind, our mind in turn, also impacts our physical form. In the world of meditation this form of comprehensive understanding is referred to as body sensing.

Think of the last time you were happy. In addition to feeling mentally excited, how did you feel on a physical level? Were you in pain? Did you find it difficult to move? Or did you feel uneasy for some reason?

Odds are you didn't feel any of this – why? When you are happy and relaxed, you don't feel physically unwell. In fact you tend to feel lighter and more physically relaxed. At the same time, the exact opposite happens when you are dealing with some sort of emotional upset. You might feel nauseous or uneasy when you're freaking out before a major exam, for example. Or, maybe you tend to feel lethargic when you are depressed or dealing with huge amounts of mental stress. Your body is a reflection of your mind. If you feel happy, your body is also happier and you are more at peace. Whereas, when you are distressed, your physical form tends to manifest in a way that reflects that negativity.

When you decided on your essentials, you made a list of what was non-negotiable for you. That list contains the most important things in your life, your bottom line. You also made the conscious decision to let go of emotional baggage and mind clutter that no longer serves you. In doing that, you eliminated stress. We can now work on removing it from other areas.

Stress comes from mental and emotional strain caused by unfavorable or challenging circumstances. Sometimes a little stress can be good for us. It can push us to try harder or improve upon ourselves. When we are attempting to live a more mindful life, stress is not in the equation. Eliminating all the stress we can is detrimental to our health and well-being, and must be done in order to live mindfully. Now is the time to make yourself, and your stress level a priority in order to keep this journey less complicated. Nothing can be done thoroughly and efficiently under stress, and making others aware of your intentions is one way of bringing down your stress level.

Sometimes, your friends and family are a source of stress for you simply by being in your life, because their stress can become your own. You have to decide that you will not let their troubles become a source of agitation for you. It is possible to be comforting and understanding without taking on other people's problems. If you are eliminating stress, the first worries to go need to be those of others.

You are not able to change their circumstances by feeling emotional strain. It has never worked, and it never will. So let the stress of others go. When you are approached with another person's stressful situation, take the time to acknowledge what they are sharing with you, and let them know that their feelings are important. If a way to eliminate their stress comes to mind, share it with them, if you like.

Let them know that you hope the best for the matter, and treat them with kindness. If you find that their troubles come back to your thoughts, recognize that this is simply you feeling empathy, and let them know that they are on your mind. Maybe you can even ask how things are, and if they have resolved the matter.

Keep yourself from actually feeling the stress, because it could possibly help them more in the long run, anyway. Your mind free from stress works more efficiently, and with all of the decluttering you have been doing, perhaps you will come up with a viable solution to their problem. Eliminating stress has a ripple effect, just like a lot of the other things you have learned thus far.

Now we are back to self. One of the most prevalent causes of stress in human beings is finances. Some would say money is the root of all evil. I say it is the bane of peace; but only if you allow it to be. Take most of the stress surrounding finances out of the equation by making everything you can automatic. We live in an amazingly effortless time where automated systems and paperless billing are commonplace. Wherever you are financially right now is what you are working with, so just make as many of these financial responsibilities as little a part of your everyday life as possible. Work with your financial institution and others to set up all that you can to be automatically deposited, paid, withdrawn, and recorded. Designate one day a week to check into things to be sure they are in good working order, but don't keep this plan in your daily thoughts. Write the weekly financial check down on your schedule like you have learned, so that you truly remove this part of the stress of finances from your thoughts until it's time to address them. Getting your finances in order, and putting the responsibilities associated with them in a safe place to be revisited takes the thinking out of it for the most part, and gets rid of that portion of stress.

Another source of stress is the everyday, mundane tasks that do not deserve the amount of significance they get. Back to the idea of auto-pilot, what other routine things can be put in that mode? Ask yourself how you can eliminate stress for each part of your day simply by taking the guess work and over-thinking away. How does your day begin? What can you put on auto-pilot?

As you prepare yourself to practice meditation, one of the things you are going to want to ensure is that you are working on your ability to understand what your body is saying to you. The easiest way to do this is by practicing body sensing. Body sensing not only allows you to control your central nervous system and allow your mind to achieve a deeper form of mental and physical relaxation, it is also known to boost your body's natural resilience. This work will help develop your ability to experience a more solid and constant sense of wholeness and well-being, in a manner unattached to your external obstacles.

Emotional Focus

As you prepare to embark on your meditative journey, another factor that you are going to need to look into is Emotional self focus. One of the core objectives of meditation is to promote self-care. In fact, meditation itself is known to have extremely therapeutic properties. Emotion focused therapy is actually a short-term psychotherapy approach that is commonly included in most meditative guides. The logic applied here is simple - emotion focused meditations are meant to identify, and cull the innate emotions the participant has. This form of the elimination of a specific emotion may be problematic to a person's growth and development, since eliminating a specific emotion in its entirety can cause people to develop mental blocks.

Research has shown that emotion focused therapy helped participants identify with their own self, which in turn allowed them to better manage their emotional experiences. Mental health issues such as depression, complex trauma etc. have shown improvement when associated with emotion focused meditations, which is why it has been used specifically to help individuals with the internalized stigma of sexual orientation, for example

As you practice using the provided meditative guides, it is important that you focus on trying to attain a specific goal during the meditative process. This ensures that you are focusing on self-care and self-awareness. As you grow up you will find that it is much easier to focus on the needs of other people rather than those of your own. However, even though this is commonplace, simply put it is not right. Remembering your own needs and feelings is just as important as tending to those of others. Furthermore, it is equally important that you ensure that your self-sacrificing mindset doesn't lead to you suppressing your own emotional needs and depriving yourself of the help that you require.

Meditation can only help you once you have begun to consciously focus on your own wants and needs. Keep in mind that the goal you set for yourself is an important part of your personal meditation. By using your meditative goals and manifesting empathy, you have the ability to attune yourself to the needs of others. But this ability can only truly manifest when you have come to terms with your own needs and have accepted yourself for who you are. Once you start to take care of yourself better you'll be better equipped to take care of others as well.

You deserve to be happy, and are a good person. These are the thoughts that you need to live by.

Identifying and Dealing with Bodily Pain

Another important factor to prepare for a meditative lifestyle, is clarity in terms of what you are working towards. Let's say for instance you are working toward dealing with physical pain. You are going to need to know specifically what kind of pain you are trying to deal with. Understanding the basis and depth of your pain will help you choose which meditative guides are going to be most effective for you.

When it comes to dealing with bodily pain, it is important that you make it a point to understand which pain management technique would be best suited for your ailment. Body-scanning allows an individual to mentally "x-ray" their body, identify their points of pain and then address or heal them as they go.

91

Another important form of pain management meditation is the mindful-movement technique. This technique teaches individuals to use mindful-movements, such as standing in a specific posture and then proceeding to go through a list physical actions, including rotating your hands and shoulders, stretching your arms, and breathing in and out at specific intervals. This type of focused breathing is another common pain management technique that can assist individuals with relaxation issues and chronic pain.

Physical Distractions

In addition to all of this, there are also a multitude of issues that you are going to want to avoid if you wish your meditation to go smoothly. For starters you're going to want to ensure that you have the proper set-up. This starts with the space where you have chosen to practice your meditation. Other factors to consider include the surrounding ambient noise, or your viewpoint from that physical space. So, always try to ensure that you have chosen a calm, empty space where you can minimize interruptions and allow yourself to relax. If you can, try to get some time outside, or at least make sure your space is well ventilated so that you have fresh air before or while you are meditating. The more fresh air you let in, the easier you will find it is to project yourself outside of the four walls you are constantly crammed in.

Begin this process by detaching yourself from any external stimuli. Turn off your phone before you embark on your meditative session. Although it is understandable that detaching yourself from social media or your phone can be difficult, particularly if you are a parent, putting in the extra effort to ensure that your children are in a safe place while you take 30 minutes for yourself is well worth it. In fact, that in itself is one of the reasons why early mornings are often considered to be an ideal time to meditate. Not only is it more than likely that you will be free of any external commitments, it is also generally a quieter time of the day.

Soft tranquil beats and musical rhythms, such as ambient music or simple instrumental tracks work well for creating a relaxing space. There are also meditative tracks and music selections available online at popular streaming sites. These are specifically composed to help add an additional level to your meditative depth.

Building Focal Points

Another extremely important part of the meditative process is finding your mind's true intent. Generally, meditation practices ask you to set an intention prior to beginning any session. This allows you to fully appreciate and utilize your meditative time. You can pre-program your meditative focus or intent by using a mental questionnaire process. Start by asking simple questions, like 'Why am I meditating?', 'What do I hope to gain from meditating?', 'What is my purpose?', 'Who am I?', 'What do I want to be?', 'How do I get where I want to be?' etc.

The idea here is to use the question to center yourself before you start meditating, so that your meditation focuses on that specific point. This is similar to how compasses show you true north, with a magnet constantly bringing the arrow back to it. Keep in mind that meditation does not have to be religious. Although certain people meditate in order to experience God, and to build on that consciousness, belief in a higher power does not increase your ability to meditate. Meditation can also be about you finding the proper wavelength for your thoughts and experiences. Is important to keep in mind, however, that although focused meditative instruction may seem superfluous, your meditative energy depends on the mind-set that you begin the meditative guide with. Taking time out to focus on your intention will not only help increase the efficiency of your meditative guide it will also help you maximize on this time you are taking for yourself.

Meditative Breathing Techniques

While there are multiple meditative breathing processes and practicing, for the purposes of this brief guide, we will be concentrating on five specific techniques that allow you to better induce meditative focus; they are Shamantha, Nadi Shondhana, Zuanqi, Khumbaka Pranayama and Box Breathing.

Shamantha is a Buddhist breathing technique that teaches you to breathe in your natural rhythm. Generally, Shamantha breathing is known as the "reset breathing" technique, because it is meant to help you come back to the present moment. In order to practice Shamantha breathing you need to first relax your body, and stretch out your spine. As you do, you are trying to find a still spot to focus your attention – that point is your focus, and it is where all your breath travels to and where it comes back from. As you focus your breathing you start to allow the natural rhythm of your breathing to course through your body, and like a rudderless boat in open seas, you simply relax and allow yourself to ride each breath as it travels through your entire body, and back out. Focus only on your breathing. Even as you wander off to different thoughts, your breathing continues to bring you back like an anchor. Shamantha breathing has been shown to help deter age-based cognitive decline, and as such is one of the best breathing techniques to use while practicing meditation.

The next form of meditative breathing that is favored by practitioners is the Nadi Shondhana technique. This type of breathing is used as a purifying technique that originates from Hinduism. This meditative practice allows your body to find its inner balance by using controlled source breathing. Nadi Shondhana is known more widely as Alternate Nostril Breathing, where each side of the nostril is blocked while the other is used to breathe for a certain period of time to assist in the smooth flow of airflow. Each side is blocked for about thirty seconds to a minute each, and the body is taught to breathe through just one nostril at a time. The exercise generally lasts for about fifteen to twenty minutes, and doing so can help reduce high levels of blood pressure and help improve reactiveness. The breathing technique is particularly well known for allowing both hemispheres of the brain to get a physical and mental workout and can help with activities that require left and right motor senses to align.

Zhuanqi originates from Taoism and is a soft breathing technique that helps the body to harmonize with nature and their surroundings. The objective of Zhuanqi is simple. By uniting your breath in mind you continue to breathe in and out, until your breathing has reached a gentle consistency. For beginners, the trick to understanding whether or not you are properly practising Zhuanqi is to notice when your breathing has gone absolutely quiet. Start by finding yourself a comfortable position, straighten your back and close your eyes, and as you do mentally focus your view on the tip of your nose. Carefully breathe in and out through your abdomen until you can hear your breathing start to quiet down. Your abdomen should be moving deeply outward with each breath that is drawn and inward as you expel the breath. As you do so, try to keep your diaphragm as still as possible, and repeat.

Khumbhaka Pranayamas, better known as the Antara and Bahya are two Hinduism inspired breathing techniques melded together to form what we refer to as intermittent breathing. The Khumbhaka Pranayamas are best practiced in an upright sitting position or alternatively in a standing posture. Prostate positions, or laying down are not advisable due to the nature of the exercise. To begin, expel all of the existing air in your lungs and then proceed to carefully inhale with your mouth until your lungs are once again full. In between breaths, once the air has been drawn in, hold the air in your lungs and after a brief pause begin to slowly release the breath. After emptying out your lungs, instead of automatically drawing in your next breath abstain for about 3 to 4 seconds. This is known as Bahya; this short deprivation will allow you to breathe in deeper and hold your breath longer, as the cycle repeats.

The Box Breathing technique uses a combination of slow breaths, and is predominantly practiced to relieve stress or anxiety. Unlike the other meditative breathing techniques mentioned here, Box Breathing, also commonly known as four-square breathing, can help regulate multiple pulmonary diseases including COPD or chronic obstructive pulmonary disease, and asthma. Similar to the Khumbhaka Pranayamas, you begin the process by expelling the excess air from your lungs and drawing in fresh air. However as you draw in air, you breath to a slow count of four. You then hold your breath for four seconds, and then finally release the breath to the count of four before repeating the process.

Seating and Posture

We will start by discussing the five basic meditative postures. Your job is to identify which posture works for you in most situations and try to stick to it. While certain meditative practices do require you to follow a specific meditative posture, most of them can be adapted to alternative postures as well.

Chair Meditation

Because most of us tend to work 9-to-5 jobs, realistically speaking we do tend to spend most of our time seated in an office chair of some sort. Chair meditation is a great way to break your midday monotony without ever having to leave your station. For seated meditation, you're going to want to straighten your back and ensure that you are touching the floor with your feet. Ideally your knees should be bent at a 90-degree angle, and your back should be as straight as possible. If you're not sure what you want to do with your hands, try simply resting them on your knees.

Standing Meditation

Sometimes you want to get out of your chair, and may be more comfortable trying a standing method. You're going to want to start by standing so that your feet are at your shoulder length apart. Bend your knees slightly, and allow pressure of your entire day to ease out through your body all the way down to your feet. As you do so adjust your hands so they are placed gently across your stomach, so that you can feel every breath that moves through your body as you embark on your personal mission.

Cross-legged Meditation

Another posture you can explore if you feel comfortable, is the traditional Indian cross-legged sitting posture. This particular posture is actually the most commonly recommended posture from meditative activities, The idea is to keep your legs crossed under each other, with your hips elevated slightly higher than the heels of your feet. If you are new to meditation, it is generally recommended that you try this posture with a cushion or a towel or some sort of soft surface underneath you so that you don't hurt yourself, since it can be difficult to hold if you are not used to it. If you feel there's too much pressure on your heels, try bringing one of your legs across the other so that the ankle of one is positioned on top of the knee of the other leg. You could alternatively bring full heels across the thighs of the opposite leg in what is commonly known as the Lotus position.

The Burmese position is slightly different in that you don't cross your legs. Instead, you can position your feet so the ankles of each foot are bent inward and facing towards the pubic area – this posture is generally preferred by those individuals who find it difficult to cross their legs.

Kneeling Meditation

If you want to keep your spine straight but don't feel comfortable crossing your legs, another great alternative is to kneel. Traditionally, this is known as the Virasana or the Vajrasana. Here you start by bending your knees and resting your body weight along the length of your shins. Your ankles should be tucked under your bottom. For ease and comfort you can opt to insert a rolled yoga mattress or a tube of some sort between your bottom and your knees.

This particular position is customarily easier than the cross-legged position, and is also generally pain-free, so your ankles will thank you.

Horizontal Meditation

If however none of these positions suit you, or you are trying a sleep inducing meditation, you will find that the posture of choice is generally the horizontal posture. As you lay down, be careful to ensure that your feet are parted at shoulder length, similar to the standing meditation posture, and your arms are laying at your sides instead of folded across your body. If you find this posture uncomfortable, you can bend your knees and elevate your hips slightly to help adjust yourself.

Chapter 8. - Techniques of guided meditations for sleep anxiety

The Storm

Welcome to this session to help you through high amounts of stress and anxiety.

Take some deep breath in through your nose and exhale out from your mouth....

Breath in....visualize what makes you anxious....and breath out watching it disappear....

Now visualize yourself standing in a big field, and no one else is around... Everything is calm and peaceful... You are surrounded by nature... notice the beauty all around you... here you are fully relaxed.

In this visual, we are going to face a very strong and powerful storm representing anxiety to make ourselves stronger within.

In the distance you see some clouds closing in as the sky grows a little darker... a storm is forming, and you feel some rain drops begin to fall...

Imagine that this storm represents your stress... it could be a mild stress with just some rain and a little wind.......... or it could be a very high stress with extremely strong winds and a very heavy rain, pouring down.

So, as you feel the storm getting even stronger and the wind is blowing harder, you remain in the meadow, completely unfazed by it.

The storm cannot hurt you here, you simply experience, and observe it.

You have a choice to react to this storm with fear... or with love and compassion. Know that this storm is harmless. This is simply a visualization you are creating........

Anxiety is our reaction to fear, worry, and even high demands...

Whether the fear it's real or not, it is best to learn the skillful reaction to all these things.

Sometimes you feel out of control and anxiety will take over in a matter of seconds, so we must handle it properly or it will handle us.

Just like sitting through the storm in the field, anxiety cannot harm you if you know that it eventually passes by.

What matters is your own reaction to the events around you.

Really embrace your anxiety now and fully let it exist -without fighting it.

You see this storm of anxiety is very dark, the clouds are raining down with fury.

You decide to slowly start walking towards it, without fear, nor worry......... just pure confidence that you are completely safe and in control......... You get closer and closer, the storm draws near and the wind blows with tremendous speed....... Yet the winds and rains have no effect on you, it is really easy for you to step forward into the wind... only your clothes are flapping in the high winds.

As you look forward you see the eye of this storm, and around that eye the winds and the rain are extremely powerful and strong, yet you have zero worry as you step inside of this eye.......

You are standing now inside this center, and everything is calm and peaceful here. You look around from within the eye of the storm and can see all the chaos around you.........but inside here its calm and bright.

This is your space......... your safe spot... and so when the stress has fully taken over you, you have a choice to let it blow over without a fight, just sitting right in the middle of it...... realizing that it cannot hurt you as you wait for it to pass.

Witness your body is the center, and any stress is just a storm surrounding you that comes and goes.

You are in control and can always come back to your safe space.

Now you feel the storm is losing its power... dying down... the rain is easing up... You see the clouds drifting away as the sky gets brighter......The sunlight peeks though the clouds then eventually comes out with great intensity, shining a brilliant light all around you.........

The anxiety has passed.

Everything is beautiful now.........This moment represents you being in a confident state of mind where stress had no control of you as it passed you by. You made it through anxiety.

Very good.

Use this session or technique whenever you find yourself in a high anxiety situation, and you will be amazed at how you can ride out the storm of stress!

Whenever you are ready, open your eyes feeling powerful and ready to take on life's challenges.

Peaceful Meadow

Hello and welcome to this relaxing session to ease anxieties and calm your stresses.

Hypnosis is a wonderful tool that allows you to relax your mind, allowing for great changes to occur deep within you.

Make sure you are very relaxed and positioned in a way where all of your muscles can let go and rest.

Let your eyes wander around, looking at your surroundings... notice the colors and textures around you... whatever you see or don't see is perfectly fine... there is no right or wrong way to do this... now allow your eyes to find something to fixate on, somewhere comfortable in front of you... whatever you are looking at, notice the color... the texture, the size or shape... take a big deep breath in and as you breathe out, close your eyes... when you inhale deeply again, open your eyes and find that same spot... exhale, closing your eyes... repeat this 3 more times, then let your eyes naturally close...

Breathing in...eyes open... breathing out... eyes closed...

Breathing in...eyes open... breathing out... eyes closed...

Breathing in...eyes open... breathing out... eyes closed, and keep them closed.

You will notice how relaxed your eyelids feel and how comfortable they are being closed.

Take a nice deep breath in and cultivate a flow of relaxation as you breathe out...

Breathe in drifting and floating into comfort... breathe out... relaxing...

Take another deep breath and let it go... in a moment I want you to imagine that there is a warm and soft blanket covering your feet... as this blanket covers you, it deeply relaxes every part that it touches... your feet feel deeply relaxed imagining this cozy blanket on your feet...

The blanket is now covering your knees and lower legs, relaxing them... thinking only of letting go of all tension...

Notice the gentle flow of your breath... your comforting blanket is now covering your entire lower legs... deeply relaxing them... allow the blanket to cover your hips... everything below your waist is released of any tension as this soft blanket covers you...

Your beautiful blanket is making you feel so carefree and loose... as the blanket sensation goes over your abdomen and belly, your muscles are becoming limp and relaxed... all worries and stresses are melting away... you are floating into a dreamy state of relaxation...

Imagine the soft blanket is covering your entire torso, along with both of your arms... it is so comfortable and soothing... feeling calm and serene... safe and warm... you don't even want to move...

Allow this enjoyment to travel up your neck all the way to the top of your head...

Your whole body is resting... feel this deep relief that you've generated all by yourself...

Pay attention to how you feel right now... do you notice any anxiety present? I bet not... It is hard to be anxious when you are this relaxed...

I will count down again from 10 and with each number I say I want you to imagine that you are descending down a flight of golden stairs... this is the stairway of relaxation, each step you take doubles your relaxation....

So begin stepping down these brilliant stairs... 10... doubling your relaxation

9... feeling even more relaxed... 8... 7... noticing the brightness of these beautiful stairs... 6... doubling the relaxation... 5... 4.... 3... so very calm... 2... extremely relaxed.... And 1... you are now a thousand times more relaxed...

Now let your mind drift and float... begin to imagine you are in a beautiful meadow....No one's around you...it's peaceful here...relaxing...feel the sun on your skin, nourishing you... the warm, soft grass under your feet...

Feel how you are finally freeing yourself from all that anxiety and stress... you feel brand new.... recharged... rejuvenated.... lighter....

Now take in all the positive vibes of this scenario...the sunlight, the calming nature surrounding you, the warm green grass under your feet...

the rhythm clouds forming and drifting away in the sky leading you to release these anxious feelings that you truly do not need...

You are now the higher version of yourself... free to be confident in all situations... with a new and improved positive attitude... living out the rest of your life with powerful intentions... authentic positivity and deep peace.....

Bring your hand into prayer position and notice how you feel...how your mind and spirit are now back on track... balanced.

Take a deep breath and bring the thought of this meadow into every day of your life... You've brought yourself complete peace of mind by simply listening to this audio and using the power of your imagination.

Say to yourself, Thank you, and experience gratitude for this moment.

Whenever you are ready, gently open your eyes, seeing the beautiful world around you... The next time you feel anxiety, remember this beautiful meadow and allow the power of your thought to relax you.

Clearing Anxieties Held in the Body

Hello, welcome to this relaxing healing body scan session, allowing you to eliminate any anxious residue that may have gotten stuck in your body.

Make sure to adjust your body so that you are in a very comfortable position, preferably lying down.

Take a deep breath in... and as you exhale, let your eyes gently close.

Now I'd like for you to focus on the sensations at the top of your head. Imagine that a gentle wave of relaxation is about to make contact with the top of your head. This relaxation eliminates all stress and fear.

Allow this relaxation to move across your forehead, melting away any anxiety you have held here...

This relaxation removes any doubt that has made its way into your brain... feel your mind letting go of despair...

Now notice your lower back and how it presses against the surface you are on, and if you feel any tension you have held here, feel the deep relaxation melting it away...

Feel the relaxation in your pelvis and hips... notice any sensations related to fear you are having there. This takes you deeper into a state of relaxation, which heals you.... letting go of these fears once and for all...

Now lets go back up the body, the same way we came, but this time imagine that in through your feet you are pulling in the energy of mother earth below. This energy is deeply loving and has a pureness that is unlike anything you have ever experienced... Imagine that this energy also carries with it your favorite color.

Imagine now, in through your feet, the feeling of love is coming in... filling you with fresh energy...

It travels up your ankles... reorganizing anything along the way... this beautiful color goes up your legs... it is so pure and so delightful... it goes all the way into your hips and pelvis... giving you confidence... making you feel centered...

Imagine the motherly energy is filling your digestive system, which is deeply healing...

See it blanketing your lower back, giving you strength along the spine...

This bright energy is going into your ribs and lungs, making you breathe passionately... each breath you take from now on is filled with love and acceptance...

See your heart being filled with the bliss of mother earth...

This new, fresh energy is traveling into your shoulders and down each arm all the way to your hands... it now allows you to take control of the choices you make with your hands... making each move you take towards health and wellness...

Feel the loving energy go up your neck and throat, opening your words to speak only your truth that lies within you. No longer do you feel pressured to say things you do not mean, or agree when you do not.

Your voice is strong and powerful, it can move mountains.

Now, feel the loving motherly energy fill your entire head... making your thoughts 100% pure...

You are a new and fresh you... you have put in the work here today to reorganize every cell in your body and every wave of energy into pure love and truth.

Good...

You are now ready to take on life, unfazed by things that once stopped you...

Chapter 9. - Learning to drop thoughts effortlessly

With concerns regarding mental health arising, you will soon find that the major players such as fear, despair, and negativity all tend to stem from the same root factor - stress. Meditation has a wonderful ability to help in stress management. Not only does guided meditation allow you to help build your mental resilience, it is also an extremely effective tool to help relax your body and mind on a more immediate basis.

Stress relief meditation, in particular, can be used not only to help improve your mental state of being but also to help you release the physical tension you feel in your own body due to anxiety.

Meditative Guide to Help with Stress Relief

In this particular form of meditation, we will be dealing with finding a way for you to release your inner struggles, your worries, your sorrows, and your stress. To begin, you want to create a peaceful atmosphere around yourself. Surround yourself with dim lights, set your room to a comfortable temperature, and, if you choose, light a candle or set out essential oils to help bring forth a calming aura.

You are now ready to start your meditative guide.

Before you close your eyes, look closely around you, and make a careful mental note of the things you see. Once you are done, close your eyes and focus on a fixed point in your mind's eye. Then, purge yourself of negativity and negative thoughts by carefully breathing in to the count of five, holding your breath until the count of four, and then releasing to the count of three.

Breathe in.

Hold.

Release.

Breathe in.

Hold.

Release.

Breathe in.

Hold.

Release.

With your eyes closed, focus your mind on the sounds that you hear around you. Look past these sounds, and beyond them, you will find the voices of the people you love most dearly. Your loved ones and your well-wishers are all gathered here around you in a circle, amidst which you are seated.

The sounds you hear around you are slowly morphing into the voices of the people you love.

Breathe in.

Hold.

Release.

Focus on the voices – the voices are talking to you.

As you do so, start to identify the fears that are holding you in place. What scares you? What intimidates you? What do you fear?

Mentally assign a bold color to each of these fears and color them in so that you can see how strong their hold on you is.

Breathe in.

Hold.

Release.

See the colors swarm you and intertwine with the other – fear into insecurity, insecurity into greed, greed into falsehoods, and so on and so forth.

As you do start to focus on the voice once again, try to hear what they are saying.

Breathe in.

Hold.

Release.

Notice that they are reminding you of your worth.

You are good.

You are kind.

You are loved.

You are needed.

You are cherished.

You are wanted.

Breathe in.

Hold.

Release.

Every voice is manifesting in the form of a bright white light that is blasting through the bold reds, blues, and greens of your fears and is opening tiny breaks through which you can release yourself.

Breathe in.

Hold.

Release.

Remind yourself that the love and belief that they have in you is enough to set you free.

As you do this, travel through your body with your next breath and do so physically for yourself.

Breathe in.

As you feel the breath travel down through your shoulders, consciously let the tension loose, feel your shoulders flex backward, and release the weight on your shoulders as you allow the energy to flow through your entire being.

Each particle of energy is now changing from a chain to a bright searing white light which is radiating through your body.

Breathe in.

Hold.

Release.

Remind yourself of the things that are shifting inside of you as you feel the transformation take place.

You are calm and relaxed.

You are loved and respected.

You are letting go of all of the unwanted fears that hold you back and instead, you are filling yourself with stillness.

Breathe in.

Hold.

Release.

Remember that with each breath, you are releasing your concerns, and with each release, you are becoming lighter and lighter until you are but the weight of a feather adrift in the wind.

Repeat after me: I am supported and loved, and stressful situations do not scare me - they merely challenge me.

I am calm and centered, and calmness washes over me with every breath that I take.

Repeat it again, in your heart: I am supported and loved, and stressful situations do not scare me - they merely challenge me.

I am calm and centered, and calmness washes over me with every breath that I take.

Breathe in.

Hold.

Release.

As you slowly open your eyes, you will feel a physical burn shift from your shoulders and, instead of stress and pain, you will feel only thankfulness and courage.

Chapter 10. - Hypnosis for a more energized morning

Hypnosis helps you to find success because it can retrain your brain to think positively. It is natural to see the negative aspects of life. There's nothing wrong with that, and you should not feel guilty over involving thinking negatively about a situation. We all do this as humans.

These hypnosis sessions won't be the answer to getting the negativity out of your life. They will help to awaken your senses and realize the positivity that exists all around you. By consistently practicing hypnosis, you will discover that you can find the good within the bad, always looking on the "bright side" of things.

Positive Thinking Hypnosis

I want you to take your right hand and make a fist. Nothing too tight, nothing too loose. Lift your thumb and your pinkie out from the rest of your fingers, holding this hand gesture while you start to become aware of your breathing.

Take this hand now and place your right pinkie over your left nostril. Press your nose so that you can no longer breathe out of this nostril. Breathe in through your right nostril now.

Then take your right thumb and place this on your right nostril, releasing your pinkie from the other one. Now, breathe out through your left nostril. This is going to help keep you focused on breathing. Repeat this several times until you feel more relaxed. The more that you do this, the more relaxed you will feel.

As you breathe in, envision that you are breathing in positive vibes and breathing out all of the bad. Everything that you feel cycles through you just like air. The negative vibes will always fade away.

From this moment forward, each breath of fresh air will be a new positive one that you bring into your body. Each breath out will be one that helps you to let go of every regret and other negative perspectives that you are holding on to. You continue to breathe in good energy, and breathe out the bad.

Each thought you have, you will now find a way to turn into a positive one. Even neutral thoughts are one that can breed positivity. This isn't going to warp your perspective negatively. You don't have to worry about having an unrealistic perspective. You will always have an idea of what reality looks like.

You will be focused on finding the positive even in situations that seem to present the biggest challenges to you.

Each positive thought that you have is one that helps you grow an even stronger mindset. Always remember that the more that you grow positivity, the more positive outcomes that will come your way. You are focused on seeing the good in everything.

You recognize that there are two sides to every story. You will not only see one side. However, you will see that the positive side is the one that is beneficial to your overall perspective.

You continue to focus on your breathing, realizing that this is helping you to relax. The more relaxed you feel, the easier it is to be positive. You are letting go of all the tension that is being held within your shoulders. You are releasing the tension that you carry on your back throughout the day.

You start to see how even stress can be a positive thing. Stress is something that helps you to put an emphasis on the things that are the most important in your life. Stress is something that isn't fun to experience. However, knowing what it feels like helps you to enjoy the moments that you are relaxed even more. Though stress can be difficult to feel, it is a reminder when you are in a good mood of the negative feelings that you don't have to experience within that present moment.

With each breath you take, you become more and more relaxed. The calmer you are, the easier it is for you to see the positive in everything that surrounds you. As negative thoughts come into your mind, you are able to turn them around easily.

When something comes into your head that fits in with a negative perspective, you look at the way in which you can change this pattern of thinking. You are not concerned with keeping up a toxic outlook on life. There is nothing beneficial that having a negative perspective has helped you with so far in this life.

You are letting go of negative emotions. You are moving forward away from the things that have happened in your past life, and you are not letting this become something that will affect how you view your future.

Though certain things that you have experienced have caused you to question your outlook and this great world, you are highly aware that there is so much positive that you have not seen simply being there.

Think of something in your past that has happened that was challenging to deal with at that time. What is it that might have been something in which you wish you had changed?

How can you twist this thing that you might feel regret, guilt, or remorse over and turn it into a positive thing that has helped you to grow to be the person that you are now?

If you can take a past experience and turn it positive, then you can be confident knowing that no matter what might be coming your way in the future, you will always know how to twist it positive and use it to your advantage.

You recognize that many of the negative thoughts that come into your head aren't even your own. Many of the negative perspectives, harsh judgments, and toxic assumptions that you might make or have made in the past were ideas planted in your brain by those around you. You might have had toxic relationships, negative people, or unhappy individuals in your life that have created the judgments first. You might also be someone who has struggled with the many negative perspectives in our society.

You are not concerned with keeping up with these negative ideas anymore. They don't do anything except provide more anxiety to the perspective you have now that you are working so hard on building in a positive light.

You continue to become more and more relaxed, assured, and calm with your positive perspective.

By being able to twist even your most negative thoughts into something positive and useful, you have discovered that it becomes that much easier to have a clearer perspective overall. You are not blinded by the fear and anxiety that can sometimes come along with having a negative perspective.

The only thing that you are focused on is finding the truth. From there, you can twist it into something positive that will help you grow. The things that are harder to remember or live through are all things that played a huge role in the development of your character.

You are allowing positivity in your life because it is something that will consistently help you to move forward. When you are thinking positive, then more positive things will come your way. It will become much easier to achieve the things that you want.

You are going to keep up with hypnosis because you know that it will be something that will continually aid in a new perspective and a healthier outlook on life overall.

You feel your entire body relaxed now, but it is your mind that is the most at peace. The more relaxed you are, the more positive thinking you will allow in your mind. The more you exude positivity, the less you feel anxious.

You feel good knowing that it is OK to be positive. You will still see the negative side sometimes, and you will not be blind to the truth. You will be focused on taking what you can from a situation and using the most from it, helping you even further to remember what needs to be focused on the most.

You feel good about yourself, and you feel good about the world. You are hopeful for the future and no longer let one small instance define your overall perspective on even larger ideas. You feel powerful, you feel assured, and you feel prepared.

Continue to focus on your breathing as you slowly come out of this hypnosis. Remember the "thumb and pinkie" trick on the days that you might be feeling like you need it the most. Keep track of your breathing now as we count down from twenty. When we reach one, you will either be out of the hypnosis or ready to move onto others and potentially even sleep.

Finding Abundance Hypnosis

This hypnotic exercise is one where I really want you to focus on the abundance that you are going to find within your lifetime. To start, let's make sure that our breathing is in perfect rhythm. Find a comfortable position and don't allow any distraction in the room in which we will be conducting this hypnosis.

We are going to be breathing in "threes." What this means is that I am going to count to three repeatedly. Each time I change, you will switch from breathing in and breathing out. Keep your hand in front of your mouth for the first few. This will be so that you can feel the air that comes out of your body.

Breathe in for one, two, three. Breathe out for one, two, three. Again, breathe in for one, two, three, and out for one, two, three.

In, one, two, three.

Out, one, two, three.

In, one, two, three.

Out, one, two, three.

You can place your hand down. Continue this breathing in for one, two, three, and out for one, two, three. In, one, two, three. Out, one, two, three.

The point of feeling your breath is for a physical reminder of your strength and your power. Without even putting effort into it, you are continuing to keep your breathing rhythm each and every day.

Now, let us move on to visualization. Picture your dream home. Whatever it might look like, envision that you are standing right in front of it. Maybe it is in a penthouse in the heart of New York. Perhaps you prefer a cabin in the middle of nowhere.

Now step toward this dream home. Walk up the stairs and into the front door. As you open the door, you discover that it is filled with the most amazing decorations that you could ever have imagined. The living room has a large TV that you can watch your favorite movies and shows on. You move into the dining room and see a massive table that is big enough to hold every last one of your friends.

You move into the kitchen, where you see pantries and cupboards filled with goodies, snacks, and other types of foods that you can have whenever you want. The floor is clean and smooth beneath your feet. The walls are clean and have pictures of those you love and who love you. You have unique art that no one else does, and everything about this home reminds you of the abundance that is present in your life.

Now you move upstairs, where you see an incredible closet. It is filled with your dream clothes and things that you never thought you would have been able to afford. You walk into the master bathroom and see that there is a large tub. There is also a separate shower that you can use whenever you want.

Continue to focus on your breathing throughout this visualization. Notice how it feels to have all these amazing things in front of you

This is a reminder that achieving all these things is entirely possible. You can find abundance in your life; you just have to know the right places to start looking.

This is the end goal that you have in mind. Starting right now, you are going to consistently create a plan to get you the things that you want. When you are feeling discouraged, come back to this house. When you are lost, come back to this house. When you feel alone, tired, anxious, stressed, and like you simply want to walk away from it all, take yourself to this house instead.

It will be a consistent reminder of all the incredible things that you still have to look forward to. The best way to find abundance like this is to find the passion deep within you to start on the path toward this success.

What is it that you can pull out from within your character that will act as a driving force as you move toward your goals? What are the things that you are concerned with the most?

Having this abundant representation at the end of this journey is going to help be the driving factor that keeps you moving forward. Once again, raise your hand to your mouth. Feel the air that comes out. If you are able to breathe, you can do anything. If you can think, you can do anything. If you can get from point A to point B, you can do anything.

The air on your hand is going to be a visual reminder of what you are capable of. Even when you aren't trying to do much at all, you are making magic within your body. Your mind is a vast nest of great ideas and important thoughts to help you be the unique individual that you are.

Abundance is possible for you. The most important part is knowing where to start and that you have done. You will continue to think about all the things that you desire and how you are going to achieve these things. Always remember your breath and this dream house as you go along your journey.

This hypnosis is going to end as we count our way down from twenty. Make sure that you always keep a positive mindset, and your wildest dreams are sure to come true. Once the hypnosis ends, you will either drift asleep or move on with your day.

Highly Successful Habits

In order to be a highly successful person, you have to make sure that you are sticking to some highly successful habits. It can be easy to fall into a pattern of negative habits that lead us to do the same things over and over again.

This meditation is going to help you remind yourself of the beneficial habits that you need to include within your life and give you the right mindset to start incorporating these habits in your everyday life.

This meditation is going to be a little different from the others. It will be presented using statements of affirmation. Repeat the meditation if you would like, or simply let the thoughts flow through your mind as if they were your own. Focus on your breathing, find a quiet place, and let your mind be guided by this meditation for successful habits.

Meditation for Successful Habits

I am a successful person. I know this because I do not measure success by how much I have done but by the choices I have made. I have made a choice to be a successful person who allows successful habits in my life.

I feel how powerful my body is all on its own. I can feel my heart pumping blood throughout my body. I see the veins on my skin that are everywhere like roots on a tree. These are parts of my body that keep every limb alive.

I can feel my brain constantly processing new emotions, new thoughts, and new ideas. I feel my brain analyzing the deepest thoughts that I have and figuring out the most challenging questions that I might face. I feel my brain trying to pick apart what it is that has led me to think a certain way. I can feel my brain processing and trying to better understand some of my most complex emotions.

Most importantly, I feel my lungs working to bring air into my body and exhale it. My body knows how to use this source of life that is all around me. When I hold my breath, my body will feel uncomfortable and make sure that I start to breathe once again.

When I count while I breathe, this makes it easier to regulate my breathing. I focus on breathing in and out by counting in patterns of five. This keeps me focused on nothing other than the way that I breathe.

I breathe in for one, two, three, four, and five. I hold my breath for a moment, feeling how powerful this air can be. I let it out for one, two, three, four, and five.

I continue to breathe in and out in this fashion, allowing each breath that I take to be one that fills me with good energy and positive vibes. I cannot deprive my body of oxygen. This is one of the most important things that I need to ensure I consistently give to my body.

Healthy and regulated breathing is just one kind of habit that I include in my life for success. My healthy habits start the moment that I wake up every single morning.

I make sure that I get out of bed at a decent time. I give myself plenty of time to prepare for this even—meaning that I always wake up earlier than I have to. I give myself time to relax even in the morning after waking up so that I can start my day with the calmest attitude possible.

I make my bed so that I have something fresh to come into at night. I also make my bed so that it is less tempting to crawl back in. I clean up my room so that I can move on from the night and focus instead on starting my day off in the healthiest way possible.

I get ready, ensuring that I brush my teeth, fix my hair, wash my face, put on all the things needed to smell good, and prepare a fresh and exciting outfit day after day. This all helps me to feel my best. I know that I don't need anything cosmetic, but I choose to make sure that I look good so that others can see how good I feel as well.

The way I look won't play a role in my success, but the way I feel about the way that I look will. Others will notice when I am not confident. Others can see some of the times that I'm insecure, but they won't always view my insecurity. My positive attitude, happy smile, and confidence are all things that make me attractive, and that is what I care about most—not the vanity aspect.

I make sure to give myself a balanced and complete breakfast. It is easier to just walk out the door with something hand-held, but giving myself time to sit down and enjoy my breakfast is a great way to start the day off right.

I ensure that I have something healthy and filling that will last me until lunch. I include fruits and vegetables because I know these have important vitamins and minerals to make me look and feel my best. I enjoy something to give me another boost of energy, like coffee or tea, but I know that a glass of water is most important to indulge in in the mornings as well.

All of these habits are helping me to be successful. The best way to have success throughout the day is to start it off right in the direction that will help to encourage positivity. When I can start my day off stress-free, relaxed, happy, and healthy, then that will be the support for everything else in my life.

I start my work off, whether it's a workout or my career, with a positive attitude. I avoid distractions and ensure that I get to the things that are most important right away. The faster that I can start off my morning, the faster the day will go.

I look out for my future self by doing what is most important first. I ensure that I put a lot of time and energy into doing the right thing so that I can live a happier life later on. There will always be more work to do, so I can't do it all as fast as possible.

I have a healthy way to judge what my limit is, so I know when I can do more work and when I need to take it easy and call it a day. I am always looking to get the most amount of work done as possible to make my life as easy as possible.

I take a healthy lunch break. I make sure to eat things that I prepared myself and do my best to avoid fast food and other tempting expensive restaurants for lunch. I want to focus only on providing my body with energy so that I can continue down the path of success.

I finish my work for the day, and I'm not opposed to staying a little past the hours I expected if it means staying caught up and preparing myself for the future. I check in with my goals daily to see whether I am making them or not. I adjust them accordingly and add new goals that I have reflected on and decided to accept into my routines.

I ensure that I leave my work at my workplace. Though it is important to stay dedicated to my work, I need time away to get a clear head. Too much work will lead to a stressed-out mind, and that will not be productive.

I am focused on making sure that I can separate myself from my work and stay true to who I am. I work on creating a positive identity. This will help me to understand my passions more, making it so that I can excel even further with the things that I choose to spend my time on.

When I go home from work, I focus on keeping up the same successful habits. I check in with new information in my area of passion and success, ensuring that I am up to date with all required knowledge in order to be successful in my field.

I include healthy habits as well, such as exercise, meditation, or yoga, to help keep me physically present, focused on my health, and continually manifesting success.

I ensure that I consistently spend time with people I love, whether it's family or friends, in order to find inspiration and keep my passion alive. I enjoy talking to other people, listening to their stories, and learning more about each other. This also helps us to learn about ourselves.

I spend some time doing something that I really enjoy and helps to keep me relaxed, such as watching a new movie, eating a tasty sweet snack, or taking a bath. I spend time with myself alone and enjoy what is going on around me in order to help keep me grounded in a place of comfort.

I constantly check in with myself to ensure that I am always focused on healthier habits. I know what I need to do to work on my intuition continually and grow my success.

I always remember to keep up with successful habits. The more healthy habits I can include in my life, the easier it will be for the things that I desire the most to fall into my path of success.

I am focused on this moment right now, one where I am aware of what needs to be done next in order to continue to find success. I can feel my powerful body aiding me in my breathing pattern. I can feel the air enter and then exit my body. Positive vibes surround me, and I am staying centered in reality.

I am going to count down from ten in order to help me move from this meditation back into the real world. Ten, nine, eight, seven, six, five, four, three, two, one.

Conclusion

Now that you are ready to fall asleep take a deep breath in. Exhale slowly and expel any tension that may have built up during the last few exercises.

As you settle in for sleep, you may begin to have thoughts about what you have done today or things you need to get done tomorrow. Take another deep breath and let those thoughts go with your next exhale. At this moment, all you need to do is clear your mind. Today is over and tomorrow will come whether you worry about it or not. For now, clear your mind so you can wake up strong and healthy for your duties tomorrow.

For now, I want you to draw your attention to your body. Where did you store your tension today? I invite you to focus your attention on the tension and let it go as we practiced earlier. Feel now where your body is relaxed. Take a few moments to appreciate the sense of relaxation your body is feeling at this moment and allow it to spread through your whole body from head to toes.

Before you drift off to bed, let's fill your mind with peaceful images. By promoting positive mental images, this will help you relax and can help avoid nightmares. As we begin, I would like you to visualize a place where you feel safe and comfortable. Take a few moments and imagine how the place would be.

When you have your safe place in mind, I would like you to start to relax your body again. In order to get rid of nightmares, you will need to release all tension from your body. When we are fearful, this can create tension in our body. Try to pay special attention to your shoulders, hands, back, neck, and jaw. Often times, these are areas where our tension can creep in.